Clinical Paediatrics for Postgraduate Examinations

Clinical Paediatrics for Postgraduate Examinations

A Guide to Success in the MRCP and DCH Examinations

Terence Stephenson
BSc BM MRCP (UK)
Lecturer in Child Health, Queen's Medical Centre, Nottingham

Hamish Wallace
MB MRCP (UK)
Leukaemia Research Fund Fellow in Paediatric Endocrinology,
Christie Hospital, Manchester

CHURCHILL LIVINGSTONE
EDINBURGH LONDON MELBOURNE AND NEW YORK 1991

CHURCHILL LIVINGSTONE
Medical Division of Longman Group UK Limited

Distributed in the United States of America by Churchill
Livingstone Inc., 1560 Broadway, New York, N.Y. 10036, and by
associated companies, branches and representatives throughout the
world.

First published 1991
  Reprinted 1991

ISBN 0-443-04172-5

British Library Cataloguing in Publication Data
Stephenson, Terence
  Clinical paediatrics for postgraduate examinations.
  1. Paediatrics
  I. Title   II. Wallace, Hamish
  618.92

Library of Congress Cataloguing in Publication Data
Stephenson, Terence.
  Clinicial paediatrics for postgraduate examinations: a guide to
  success in the MRCP and DCH examinations/Terence Stephenson,
  Hamish Wallace.
      p.   cm.
    ISBN 0-443-04172-5
    1. Pediatrics — Examinations, questions, etc.   I. Wallace,
  Hamish.
  II. Title.
    [DNLM: 1. Pediatrics — examination questions.   WS 18 S837c]
  RJ48.2.S74   1991
  618.92′00076 — dc20
  DNLM/DLC
  for Library of Congress   90–1793

Produced by Longman Singapore Publishers (Pte) Ltd.
Printed in Singapore

Preface

This book has been inspired by our experience both in teaching doctors for paediatric postgraduate examinations and our own experience in passing them. This book is not a short textbook of paediatrics but a guide to the clinical examination of children. The format is specifically designed to aid revision for the clinical parts of the MRCP and DCH and where possible the requirements for success in these examinations have been stated. There are, by the constraints of a book that is intended to be a constant companion, some omissions, but we have tried to cover all the areas which we consider are important.

We hope that this book will appeal not only to those paediatricians entering higher medical training but also to doctors in general and community practice who have a special interest in child health.

Throughout the book we have referred to the child as 'he'; no sexism is intended.

T.S.
H.W.

This book is dedicated to Jacqui and Amanda.

Contents

1. Introduction

The clinical examination in the second part of the MRCP exam is one of the most difficult hurdles that any paediatrician in training must face. Likewise, most candidates who fail the DCH exam do so on the clinical part. Many candidates feel that these exams are too artificial, merely test the ability to pass an exam, and are unrelated to the skills required on the ward and in outpatients. However, the exam is designed to test the basic clinical skills of using symptoms and signs to arrive at a diagnosis and is on the whole fair and not esoteric, particularly now that it is also conducted in busy provincial centres. Nevertheless, all exams are artificial and the aim of this book is to show you how to improve your technique in this unusual and demanding setting. Whilst there are many aids to passing postgraduate exams in adult medicine, there is no satisfactory guide to the clinical parts of the MRCP and DCH exams, which is why we wrote this book.

Membership of the Royal College of Physicians

To qualify for the second part of the paediatric MRCP (which is held three times a year in London, Edinburgh and Glasgow), you must have been fully registered for at least 18 months and you must have passed the first part of the MRCP (written multiple choice exam based largely on adult medicine) of one of these three United Kingdom colleges. There is reciprocity so that you do not necessarily have to sit the multiple choice exam and the clinicals with the same college.

The second part of the MRCP has both written and clinical sections, separated by about six weeks. The written exam lasts for three hours and consists of detailed case histories ('grey cases'), data interpretation and slides. The written section of the exam is marked out of 20, with a mark of 10 or more being considered a pass. Several books have already been published giving advice on this written part of the MRCP.

The clinicals for the MRCP examination consist of three parts which are marked independently of each other. They are the long case, the short cases and the oral, and they are usually conducted in this order. To make marking as fair as possible, each candidate is examined by a different pair of examiners for each of the three parts. Moreover, the examiners are not aware:

1. of how many attempts you have previously had at the clinical exam;

2. of your performance in the written exam, i.e. whether you had a borderline written paper requiring good clinicals to compensate;

3. of your marks in the other sections of the clinical exam.

Each part of the clinical section is given a mark which is agreed by each pair of examiners. A 'close marking' system is employed, with a range of 0–10, and a mark of 5 or more is a pass. By and large, a mark of 4 is correctable in all but the short cases, when no matter how many marks of 7 or even 8 a candidate may have scored in other sections of the exam, a mark less than 5 is a fail. This underlines the emphasis the Royal Colleges have put on the short cases, which are considered to be the very heart of the exam.

If a candidate was allowed to progress to the clinicals with a borderline written paper (i.e. a mark of 9 out of 20), he must gain an extra 3 compensatory marks in the clinical and oral examinations in order to pass the examination overall. Some examples are given in Table 1.1.

Table 1.1   Scoring system for the second part of the MRCP examination

Written (out of 20)	Oral (out of 10)	Clinical (out of 20)	Total (out of 50) Long and short cases combined	Result
10	5	10	25	pass
9	5	11	25	fail

The one mark dropped in the written is not compensated by one mark extra in the clinical. The result is therefore a fail

9	6	12	27	pass

The borderline written mark is compensated by the extra 3 marks in the other parts of the exam.

9	4	14	27	fail

Two sections of the exam have been failed and even an excellent performance in the long and short cases cannot make amends.

11	4	10	25	pass
10	4	10	24	fail
9	9	9	27	fail

The three parts of the clinical exam are as follows:

1. The long case is to test the ability of the candidate to take a detailed history, to perform a full systematic examination and to use the information obtained to arrive at a differential diagnosis, a problem list and a plan for management. The candidate is allowed one hour for this, and must then present his findings and interpretation in a succinct and clear manner and be able to elicit at the bedside the physical signs which he claims to have found. He may also be asked

to discuss laboratory reports and X-rays. The examiners spend 20 minutes with the candidate.

2. The short cases are where most people fail and it is principally with these in mind that this book was written. Unlike the long case, in which there is a little time in which to collect one's thoughts after examining the patient, the short cases are conducted in the presence of the examiners to allow them to assess technique. The candidate must decide quickly what is wrong with the child and it is this ability to gently, quickly and correctly elicit physical signs and rapidly interpret them which the short cases are designed to test. The time allotted for short cases is 30 minutes; usually each examiner questions the candidate for 15 minutes while the other examiner marks. A bell may sound after 15 minutes to indicate that they should change rôles, but this sequence is sometimes altered by individual examiners. The examiners aim to use the short cases to assess the candidate on at least four systems, almost always including a developmental assessment. You may be asked to examine an entirely normal child.

The examination of a short case is frequently introduced by a piece of history, e.g. the examiner might simply say, 'Look at this child and tell me what you notice' or, alternatively, 'This young girl has become cyanosed over the last few months, why do you think this might be?'. The first question is all embracing and you should refer to Chapter 13 on common exam syndromes for advice on how to cope with this type of question. However, examiners are now encouraged by the colleges to introduce the case in order that the examination bears some similarity to real clinical practice, in which a child is rarely examined 'blind'. The second type of question is therefore an invitation to show that you can examine the relevant parts quickly, as you would have to do in a busy clinic, and step outside the restraints of single system examination.

This difficult skill of 'rationalized examination' presumes as an essential prerequisite that you know the differential diagnosis of common physical signs. For example, if you do not know that the differential of a lump in the neck includes a lymphoma, you will not automatically offer to examine for hepatosplenomegaly and will be marked down compared to a candidate who does and can explain why. In order to convey this appearance of being able to 'think on your feet', we strongly recommend that you familiarize yourself with the lists of differential diagnoses we have provided in this book. These are also essential for the oral examination.

We have tried throughout the text to suggest a method for approaching a child with a common symptom or sign which allows you to examine the relevant parts in the most efficient way. This is how experienced doctors work in practice. This method stems from considering the differential diagnosis of

that symptom or sign and then looking for or excluding other physical signs and thereby narrowing the differential. However, it is clearly impossible for us to cover every case which might arise in a postgraduate paediatric exam (see Tables 1.2–1.4 for a list of cases seen by candidates whom we have recently taught), and this book is therefore about form as much as content. Perfect the habit of thinking through the sequence
— differential diagnoses
— examine relevant parts
— exclude alternative diagnoses
— final diagnosis
so that this process is second nature even when you are confronted by a situation which we have not covered.

We have selected the 'common' short and long cases at the end of each chapter from our own experience of organizing clinical exams. Obviously, most of the children are requested to attend some time in advance so they are likely to be children with chronic diseases and signs which do not fluctuate. However, a child with a long and complex history and virtually no

Table 1.2 Typical long cases recently encountered in the clinical part of the MRCP examination

Down's syndrome with a ventricular septal defect
Ulcerative colitis
Newly diagnosed diabetic
A chromosome deletion syndrome
Hydrocephalus
Neurofibromatosis
Cystic fibrosis
Marfan's syndrome

Table 1.3 Typical short cases in the clinical part of the MRCP examination

Mitral stenosis
Acute arthritis
Pneumonia
Hepatosplenomegaly
Developmental assessment of a normal 3-year-old
How old is this child (2 years)?
Tracheostomy for congenital haemangioma
Optic atrophy
Café au lait spots
Ventricular septal defect
Osteogenesis imperfecta
Russell–Sivler syndrome
Oculocutaneous albino
Clubbing
Splenomegaly and anaemia
Hemiplegia
Portal hypertension
DiGeorge's syndrome
Henoch–Schönlein purpura

Table 1.4 Some oral topics from recent MRCP examinations

Neonatal vitamin D and calcium requirements
Management of diabetic ketoacidosis
Education of a new diabetic
Adolescent problems and diabetes
Kawasaki's disease
Mycobacteria
Petechiae in a neonate
Microcephaly
Incubation, prodromes, and infectivity of common exanthema
Stridor
Hydrocephalus and cerebrospinal fluid circulation
Malaria and kala-azar
Hookworm
Vaginal bleeding in a 3-year-old
Toddler diarrhoea, constipation and soiling
Apnoea of prematurity
Bronchopulmonary dysplasia

---

physical signs may still make an excellent long case. Finally, do not be surprised to see children with acute conditions in the exam; cases may have to be found at short notice from the wards. Moreover, the Royal Colleges have emphasized the need to make the exam a realistic test of common paediatric problems and not just a catalogue of the esoteric.

The assessment of a short case by a candidate can be made at three levels. If you are certain of the diagnosis, don't 'beat about the bush'. For example, 'This child has Von Gierke's disease'. This response scores maximum marks if you are right, but if you are wrong you get no marks for 'rough work'. So if you are less confident of your diagnosis, an appropriate statement might be 'The abnormal findings were a very large liver, palpable kidneys, doll's face and short stature. This is consistent with a glycogen storage disease.' Even if your interpretation is wrong, you will still gain marks if the physical signs are correct. Thirdly, if you cannot fit the signs together to make a diagnosis, the best approach is to list the important positive and negative findings. For example, 'There is a 10 centimetre, smooth, non-tender liver and both kidneys are also palpable.' You may then be asked to commit yourself to a diagnosis but this is better than overconfidently plumping for a diagnosis initially when the signs obviously did not fit, especially if it is the wrong diagnosis!

If you found no abnormalities, say so. Do not invent signs, as sins of commission are worse than sins of omission. Similarly, if you are not certain of a physical sign, e.g. whether a spleen is palpable, then it is better to be confident and say, 'The spleen is not palpable', rather than 'I think the spleen may possibly be just palpable'.

It is said that the more short cases you see, the more likely you are to pass. While it is true that if you are on your sixth case, you are probably doing well, the converse is not true.

Some 'short' cases are in fact very complex or involve more than one system and if you have only seen three difficult cases but got them all right, you are just as likely to pass. Most candidates fail the short cases because of a lack of technique rather than a lack of knowledge. Alternatively, they may fail because of inadequate anticipation of what type of cases to expect. This book should help with both of these pitfalls, but clearly there is no substitute for practising on the wards under exam conditions, with either a fellow candidate or a registrar taking the part of the examiner.

3. The oral examination is to test depth and breadth of knowledge and reasoning power. It lasts 20 minutes and the candidate is questioned by each examiner in turn. The usual practice is for the examiners to begin by asking general questions, often based on current topics in the medical journals.

The examiners are encouraged by the Royal Colleges to test the candidates on the management of acute situations and on their understanding of applied anatomy, pharmacology and biochemistry, and the physiological basis of disease processes. You are as likely to be asked about the physiological basis of cyanosis as about the management of acute asthma. There are always two facets to a child's problem. On the one hand, you may be asked about the investigation of a complex endocrine problem such as ambiguous genitalia, and on the other hand you may be expected to discuss sensibly the social and psychological aspects of a chronic paediatric condition such as cystic fibrosis. Child abuse is an example of the social side of paediatrics which frequently seems to come up for discussion.

However, examiners are individuals and there is no uniform schedule that they must follow, although it is recommended that each examiner covers three different subjects. Do not be afraid to say that you do not know. There is nothing more detrimental than allowing yourself to be drawn into a subject about which you know very little. No examiner expects you to know everything but some will be only too happy to plumb the depths of your ignorance. It is clearly far better to take your chances with another topic than press on with one about which you know little.

Finally, be prepared for the examiner who invites you to talk about a subject which interests you. This is a great chance to control proceedings and show how widely read you are. Examiners are advised not to persist on a subject about which the candidate shows little knowledge or, conversely, on a topic on which he is extremely well rehearsed. Some advice on oral exam technique is given in the final chapter. Again, practice makes perfect.

Diploma in Child Health   The DCH is primarily for junior doctors intending to enter general practice or as a preliminary exam for career paediatricians before they attempt the more difficult MRCP.

The examination is held twice a year and the only obligatory requirement is that the candidate is either fully registerable with the General Medical Council of the United Kingdom, or has limited registration which has not become non-renewable. At least 12 months' experience in the care of children (in hospital or in the community) is recommended but not mandatory, and we know of many candidates who have been successful after only 6 months in hospital paediatrics.

This examination also has written and clinical parts. The written part consists of two papers: paper I (3 hours) has 10 'short notes' questions and two case commentaries and paper II has 60 multiple choice questions for which 2 hours are allowed. Paper II is marked initially and candidates must gain sufficient marks in this to go forward to the clinical section. Paper I is not even marked if a candidate is eliminated due to insufficient marks in paper II. The clinical section consists of one long case and several short cases. The candidate is allowed 40 minutes for the history and examination of the long case and then spends about 20 minutes with the examiners. 25 minutes are allowed for the short cases and great emphasis is placed on developmental assessment, for which at least 10 of the 25 minutes are set aside. The short cases may be very short and we know of one candidate who saw 10 children in 25 minutes and passed! Alternatively, you may be asked to examine several aspects of one child.

Further information about both the MRCP and the DCH can be obtained from the following address:

Royal College of Physicians
11 St Andrew's Place
Regent's Park
London NW1 4LE.

2. The long case

The history in the paediatric long case is usually obtained with the help of the parents. A useful list of headings for obtaining and presenting a history is given below. The most common errors are an inadequate developmental history and an inadequate social history. Do not attempt to present the whole history verbatim; you must organize it so that you present all the positive and the important negative points in a logical sequence. The existence of a pet cat may be relevant but the fact that his name is Charlie is not!

Try to stick to the order given below, but examiners do not always ask you simply 'What is the history?' so be prepared for questions such as 'How has this child's illness affected development?' or 'What are his problems and how would you help him?' which require you to adopt a different format. Nothing will annoy the examiner more than trotting out a conventional history in response to these questions so be prepared to be flexible.

Check-list for history taking

Name —
Age —
Source of history (father/mother/other) —
Presenting complaint — use their own words. The parents may actually tell you the diagnosis.

History of presenting complaint

Obtain a complete chronological sequence of events, noting especially the mode of presentation and the timing of complications and how they have been managed. Include drugs prescribed, investigations carried out and operations performed. Deeper inquiry about important symptoms must be made regarding
— time of onset
— site
— duration
— frequency
— severity
— relieving factors
— exacerbating factors
— diurnal or seasonal variation

If the presenting complaint is a chronic one, e.g. wheezing, the history of the presenting complaint may overlap with the past medical history and duplication during presentation should be avoided.

Past medical history | Obviously, all previous hospital admissions should be catalogued. Visits to casualty, outpatients or assessment centres may be forgotten by parents so enquire about these directly. Likewise, childhood exanthema are often disregarded as being trivial:

1. Birth history
— pregnancy and gestation
— mode of delivery and birth weight
— admitted to special care and why?
If a neonatal, genetic or developmental case, more detail is required, e.g. miscarriages, terminations, stillbirths, amniocentesis, neonatal deaths.
2. Nutritional history
— bottle- or breastfed and for how long
— timing of introduction of solids/cereals
— current dietary intake if relevant to complaint of an older child
— diabetic exchanges.
3. Immunization history
— ask specifically about whooping cough vaccine and record reasons in detail for failure of uptake (you must know in detail the absolute and relative contra-indications to all immunizations).
4. Developmental history
— gross motor   know at least four milestones for
— fine motor/visual   different ages which
— speech and hearing parents can easily
— social   answer (Ch. 9).
5. Schooling
— which school and what sort?
— whether he is in a special class or has remedial help
— does he miss school? Press the parent for an estimate of this, e.g. 3 months in the last year
— how does he get on with other children?

Family and social history | Ages of parents and what they both do.
Social class (determined in this country by the Registrar-General's classification of the father's occupation).
Marital status and how long married.
Consanguinity (this is particularly common in Asian Muslim families).

Number of siblings and age range.
Family history of diabetes, atopy or fits.
Pay attention to detailed family history if a hereditary or infectious disease is involved, especially tuberculosis in a family from an ethnic minority.

Housing: type of accommodation (rented or owned, house or flat, number of bedrooms, washing and toilet facilities, heating).

Details of extended family if a chronic condition or the parents need help in looking after the child.
Document social services involvement and domiciliary support, e.g. diabetic health visitor.
Any pets at home.

Drug history

List drugs, frequency and doses (you must know why they were prescribed, what the side-effects are, and if there have been any). Parents understand 'medicines' better than the stigmatized term 'drugs', although a history of smoking or glue-sniffing should not be overlooked. In the neonate or breastfed baby, a maternal drug history is also important. Ask about allergies.

Systems enquiry

This is rarely necessary in routine paediatric history taking, unless there is a chronic multisystem disease. There are a few general questions which provide a useful 'screen' and the remainder are included for completeness.

General:
— weight loss
— appetite
— is he his usual self?

Cardiovascular:
— shortness of breath on exertion, or a baby breathless and sweaty on feeding, or slow to feed
— blue episodes
— squatting
— palpitations or chest pain
— dizzy spells or fainting (may be confused with fits)

Respiratory:
— sore throat or earache
— cough, particularly nocturnal or in relation to exercise, whether productive of sputum and clear or purulent
— wheezing; again ask if nocturnal or exercise induced
— shortness of breath, especially compared to peers during games
— frequent chest infections (as evidenced by frequent antibiotic courses from GP or previous chest X-ray)
— aspiration (e.g. history of playing with peanuts)
— haemoptysis

Gastrointestinal:
— abdominal pain
— vomiting
— jaundice
— diarrhoea or constipation (document exact frequency and appearance of stools)
— travel abroad, contacts and 'fast' foods may be relevant to infectious diseases

— blood in the stools
— pruritus ani

Genitourinary:
— stream
— dysuria
— frequency
— nocturia or enuresis (primary or secondary)?
— incontinence
— haematuria
— age of menarche

Neurological:
— fits, faints or funny turns
— headaches
— loss of smell or taste
— visual problems
— deafness or dizziness
— numbness or unpleasant sensations
— weakness, clumsiness or frequent falls
— incontinence

From the history you should have a good idea of which systems will have abnormal physical signs and therefore plan to concentrate your attention on these systems. However, there is ample time in the long case to examine every system thoroughly and this is expected. For instance, the child with developmental delay may also have an innocent heart murmur.

Be prepared to discuss the effect of the child's problems on the lifestyle of the rest of the family. In the case of a handicapped child, what special financial allowances are they entitled to, what modifications have been made to the home, and what domestic compromises have been necessary?

You will be provided with a current height and weight and you must plot these values and the head circumference on appropriate centile charts, which will be available. Leave unpleasant parts of the examination until last, e.g. examination of the ears and throat and measurement of head circumference, otherwise rapport will be lost early and never regained. Time yourself carefully so that you have at least 10 minutes remaining, after completing the history and examination, in which to organize your thoughts and formulate a differential diagnosis, a problem list and a plan for management, anticipating the development of possible medical and psychosocial complications. Consider relevant investigations, such as chest X-ray or ECG, which you might be asked to interpret.

You have not finished until you have recorded the blood pressure, looked at the child's fundi (even if you don't think it is relevant) and tested a urine sample which will be available, so know how to use dip sticks. Don't forget the centile charts and take them with you for discussion with the examiners.

3. General advice on examining children

Examining children is an art and not a science and you should rehearse the examination of individual systems and features until this is second nature. The examiner will be impressed by your efficiency and technique even if you don't get everything right. A guide to examining each of the major systems is given in the following chapters, but there are some general rules which are listed here to save duplication.

1. Introduce yourself to the child's guardian and ask if you may examine the child. Ask the child's name if you have not already been told it and talk to the child as you examine him or her.

2. Speak quietly to the child but clearly to the examiners. The hearty candidate who greets his short case with a slap on the back and a loud welcome has clearly not had much experience of examining children.

3. Warm your hands and remove a watch or rings which might scratch a child. It is unfortunately impractical to wash your hands between each short case.

4. Once you have been introduced to your case you must take control of the situation and appear at ease examining children, giving clear instructions as necessary, positioning the child appropriately and ensuring adequate exposure of the part to be examined. Undress an infant yourself and lend a hand to an older child. The candidate who stands idly by while the parent undresses the child appears to lack confidence and is missing information regarding tone, dexterity etc.

5. Never hurt a child as this can be avoided by enquiring about tenderness before laying on hands and by noting 'drip' sites, bandages etc.

6. Do not ask a toddler for permission to do something. He will almost certainly refuse! 'Can I listen to your tummy?' . . . . . . 'No'. Where do you go from here? Rather, 'I am going to listen to your tummy'. Listening to his teddy's tummy first may win round an awkward child.

7. Avoid standing over a small child by getting down to his level. If he is sitting on his mother's knees, then be prepared to get onto yours.

8. If at all possible, examine a young child in close proximity to his parent. Children of 3 or under are very reluctant to be separated from their parent by a stranger.

9. Feel free to ask the examiner or parent to distract the child with a toy if this will help you continue your examination.

Some examiners like a running commentary as you examine the appropriate system. We would advise against doing this unless you are specifically asked to as it is easy to commit yourself wrongly to a physical sign before you have the complete picture.

The technique of examining children varies with age. For older children the order outlined in the following chapters can usually be adhered to because the child is sufficiently co-operative. In the younger child, there may be interruptions to regain the child's attention and toys are a valuable adjunct. Try and examine an infant on his parent's knee and employ a more opportunistic approach. As much information as possible must be gained from inspection before the child is disturbed by undressing, by strange hands and by the hostile oroscope. The child may have to be examined in the order in which he chooses to present himself, rather than adhering to a preconceived sequence. However, although the physical signs may be elicited in this haphazard manner, the information must be organized by the candidate within a neat framework so that it can be presented in a logical fashion.

4. The cardiovascular system

The cardiovascular system can be examined systematically as described in the following sections. However, in our experience the candidate may not be invited to examine the whole system. Often you will be requested to 'feel the pulse', 'localize the apex beat' or 'listen to the heart'. Our advice is that you follow these instructions exactly, as failure to do so may antagonise the examiners.

Inspection Look at the whole child. Estimate the approximate age and judge the general health, e.g. failure to thrive, short of breath, dysmorphic features.

Face 1. Central cyanosis, best seen in the tongue, may be obvious at rest or only after exercise, such as feeding, crying or running. Cyanosis is detectable if there is more than 5 g/dl of deoxygenated haemoglobin in the skin capillaries, corresponding to an arterial saturation of about 75%. Cyanosis can therefore be present at a normal PaO_2 if there is polycythaemia, or difficult to detect if there is concomitant anaemia.

2. Syndromes to look for (see Ch. 13):

— Down's
— Turner's
— Cri du chat
— Noonan's
— Marfan's
— William's
— Edward's and Patau's syndromes are associated with congenital heart disease but are unlikely to appear in the exam.

3. Show that you know that detection of caries is an important part of outpatient follow-up by commenting on the teeth while you assess the colour of the tongue.

Hands 1. Peripheral cyanosis must be distinguished from central cyanosis.

2. Clubbing (and conjunctival injection and gum hypertrophy) indicate that the cyanosis is chronic.

3. Splinter haemorrhages and Osler's nodes in infective endocarditis (rare in exams).

4. Tuberous and tendon xanthomata of familial hypercholesterolaemia. Feel over the elbows in a child who is hypertensive.

Chest   1. Operation scars: axillary or subscapular scar from closure of patent ductus arteriosus (PDA); axillary scar from pulmonary artery banding, Blalock shunt or coarctation repair; central sternotomy from open heart surgery.

2. Asymmetry: bulge of left chest due to cardiomegaly in a thin child.

3. Harrison's sulcus: may occur in conditions with increased pulmonary blood flow.

Palpation

Arterial pulse: 1. Check that both brachial pulses are present and equal in volume. At the end of the examination test for absent or decreased femoral pulses (diagnosing coarctation). If this is difficult, palpation of foot pulses excludes coarctation. Radio-femoral delay is virtually impossible to detect in a child with coarctation.

Unequal pulses:
— classic left Blalock–Taussig shunt (absent left brachial)
— coarctation preceding or involving the left subclavian artery or flap aortoplasty repair of coarctation (decreased left brachial)
— cervical rib (either brachial absent, especially on abduction of the shoulder)
— previous cardiac catheter (radial or brachial absent)
— embolization
— congenital malformation (absent radial pulse)
Is the radius absent too?
— Holt–Oram syndrome: most have atrial septal defect (ASD)
— 'VATER' association (acronym for the constellation of vertebral anomalies, anal atresia, tracheo-oesophageal fistula): 50% have ventricular septal defect (VSD)
— Thrombocytopenia and absent radii syndrome: 25% have congenital heart disease
Assess the following, using the right brachial, which is much easier to assess than the radial pulse.

2. Rate: Always count this over 10 seconds whilst deliberately looking at your watch. Never guess at a rough figure, you may be wildly wrong.

Age (years)	Normal range (beats per minute)
0–2	80–140
2–6	75–120
>6	70–110

Bradycardia (rare short case):
— junior athletes!
— drugs (β-blockers and digoxin)
— complete heart block: all forms of heart block are rare in children. It may occur in otherwise normal children but is

usually the result of structural heart disease, intracardiac surgery or rheumatic carditis (rare nowadays).

Tachycardia:

— must be a sinus tachycardia due to an anxious child as tachyarrhythmias make very unsuitable exam cases!

3. Rhythm: regular or irregular? Regularly irregular or irregularly irregular?

Respiratory sinus arrhythmia:

— universal in young children.

Extrasystoles:

— extremely common in normal children and disappear with exertion whereas pathological extrasystoles (e.g. digoxin toxicity) are exacerbated by exertion.

Atrial fibrillation:

— irregularly irregular for rate, volume (and loudness of heart sounds). Often associated with structural defects and possibly congestive cardiac failure. Causes of atrial fibrillation are

   — atrial septal defect (ASD)

   — open heart surgery

   — Ebstein's anomaly of tricuspid valve

   — rheumatic mitral stenosis (almost exclusively immigrant children now).

4. Volume and character: assessed by palpation with the index finger of the brachial pulse or femoral in an infant.

(a) Large volume and rapid collapse = 'water—hammer pulse':

— PDA (common): often a neonatal case

— aortic regurgitation (rare)

(b) Small volume:

— low stroke volume, therefore either

   (i) pump failure (heart failure)

   (ii) shock (circulatory failure due to relative or absolute hypovolaemia)

   (iii) outflow obstruction (aortic stenosis (AS), pulmonary stenosis (PS) or pericardial effusion)

While the first two are commoner in clinical practice, it is the third group of conditions which are more likely to be seen in the exam.

(c) small volume, slow rising and sustained = 'plateau pulse':

— aortic stenosis

(d) varying volume:

— extrasystoles

— atrial fibrillation

— incomplete heart block

(e) normal volume, rapidly rising and ill sustained = 'jerky pulse':

— hypertrophic obstructive cardiomyopathy (HOCM)

(f) 'pulsus paradoxus': not a paradox at all but an exaggeration

of a normal phenomenon, i.e. the fall in blood pressure with inspiration. However, if you do detect pulsus paradoxus then you should offer to measure this by sphygmomanometry. A paradox of greater than 15 mmHg is abnormal and possible causes are:
— pericardial effusion
— constrictive pericarditis
— severe airways obstruction (asthma)
Only the last of these is common (not in exams).
Always feel quickly in the suprasternal notch for the thrill associated with aortic valve stenosis.

Assessment of jugular venous pressure is not an important part of examination of the cardiovascular system in paediatrics. It can only be measured in older children and whilst it is elevated in right heart failure, fluid overload and pericardial tamponade, none of these is likely in the exam.

Palpation of the precordium

Apex beat   The furthest lateral and inferior position at which the finger is lifted by the cardiac impulse.

1. Position: normally the 4th intercostal space, in the midclavicular line. If the position is abnormal, then clearly define this by counting rib spaces and using landmarks.
(a) displaced to left
    — cardiomegaly
    — scoliosis
    — pectus excavatum
(b) apex on right side
    — feel for the liver
    — may be true dextrocardia or dextroposition (the heart is pushed or pulled to the right, e.g. pulmonary fibrosis, diaphragmatic hernia)
    — dextrocardia with abdominal situs inversus is less likely to have other congenital cardiac anomalies
    — Kartagener's syndrome

2. Quality:
(a) sustained   — aortic stenosis
(b) forceful   — left ventricular hypertrophy
(c) systolic thrill at   — ventricular septal defect (VSD)
    left sternal edge   — atrio-ventricular (AV) canal defect
(d) parasternal heave   — right venticular (RV) hypertrophy

3. Thrills: localize the site. The accompanying murmur is by definition at least 4/6 in intensity.

4. Palpable 2nd sound: this will be the pulmonary component and reflects pulmonary hypertension.

Auscultation   Palpate right brachial with your left hand while auscultating; this will help you to time the sounds. Decide:
— is the 1st heart sound normal?
— is the 2nd heart sound normal and does it split normally?
— are there added sounds or murmurs?
— if so, in systole, diastole or both?
Listen over the apex (= mitral area) with diaphragm and then bell of stethoscope. Then use the diaphragm as follows:
— 4th intercostal space, left sternal edge = tricuspid area
— 2nd intercostal space, left sternal edge = pulmonary area
— 2nd intercostal space, right sternal edge = aortic area
If there is a systolic murmur, listen over the carotids, loud radiation here suggesting aortic stenosis.

Always listen at the back; innocent murmurs do not radiate to the back. With an older, co-operative child, always listen again along the lower LSE as he breathes out and leans forward (otherwise you may miss the murmur of aortic regurgitation). Decide what you are going to say before you take your stethoscope out of your ears!

Heart sounds   1. Loud 1st sound
— ASD
— mechanical prosthetic valve

2. Variable loudness 1st sound
— heart block
— atrial fibrillation
The 2nd heart sound is very important in paediatric cardiology. If it is of normal intensity and splits normally, many important conditions are excluded.

3. Loud 2nd sound
— increased pulmonary flow, e.g. PDA, ASD, large VSD
— pulmonary hypertension

4. Split 2nd sound
— universal in healthy children and widens on inspiration. Aortic closure precedes pulmonary closure.
— fixed splitting (no change with respiration): ASD
— widely split: ASD, pulmonary stenosis (PS), right bundle branch block (RBBB)
— reverse splitting (widens on expiration): left bundle branch block (LBBB), severe AS

5. Single 2nd sound
— Fallot's tetralogy or pulmonary stenosis (inaudible pulmonary component)

Extra heart sounds   3rd sound (after 2nd, i.e. early in diastole, low pitched):
— may be confused with split 2nd sound or opening snap

— heard best with the bell over the apex
— normal finding in healthy children
— heard if there is failure of either ventricle

4th sound (before 1st, i.e. late diastole, low pitched):
— easily confused with ejection click
— never a normal finding
— failure of either ventricle
— pulmonary hypertension

Opening snap (after 2nd heart sound, high pitched):
— mitral stenosis (very rare short case)

Ejection click (after 1st heart sound, high pitched):
— aortic or pulmonary valve stenosis (early systolic)
— floppy mitral valve (midsystolic)

Murmurs   Try to define the following parameters:
— intensity (grades 1 to 6; grade 4 if a thrill is palpable)
— where is it loudest?
— where does it radiate?
— timing (systolic, diastolic or both)
— duration (e.g. early systolic or pansystolic)
— pitch and quality (high or low; harsh, blowing or rumbling)
— change with respiration or posture (venous hum disappears on lying down with legs elevated)
Remember to listen over the back (PDA and coarctation).
The '10 S test' of an innocent murmur:
1. symptom free
2. systolic
3. short
4. soft
5. heard over only a small area
6. split 2nd sound
7. sitting/standing (i.e. varies with posture)
8. sternal depression (benign murmurs with pectus excavatum)
9. no other abnormal signs
10. special tests (electrocardiogram and chest X-ray) normal
Also, the pulses are normal and the femorals are present!
Innocent murmurs may be

— Still's murmur (early systolic at LSE)
— pulmonary ejection systolic murmur
— venous hum

Classification of murmurs   (a) Systolic murmurs: in order starting with the most common and with the sites where the murmur is heard loudest. ESM = ejection systolic murmur, PSM = pansystolic murmur.

Innocent flow murmur (ESM) — left sternal edge or pulmonary area

Anaemia (ESM)	— left sternal edge or aortic area
VSD (PSM)	— left sternal edge, 4th intercostal space
PS (ESM)	— pulmonary area, left 2nd intercostal space
ASD (ESM)	— pulmonary area, left 2nd intercostal space
Left ventricular outflow	— aortic area, right 2nd intercostal space
	— aortic stenosis (rare) or bicuspid aortic valve (relatively common) and may radiate to the carotids
	— hypertrophic obstructive cardiomyopathy (very rare)
Coarctation (PSM)	— left sternal edge and between scapulae
Mitral regurgitation (PSM)	— apex and left axilla

(b) Diastolic murmurs: much rarer than systolic murmurs. Never innocent.

ASD	— tricuspid flow murmur, low pitched over left sternal edge
VSD	— mid-diastolic mitral flow murmur with large defect
Aortic regurgitation (rare)	— high-pitched decrescendo over left sternal edge, especially in expiration
Mitral stenosis (very rare)	— low pitched at apex

(c) Continuous murmurs:

Innocent venous hum	— below either clavicle and may disappear on lying the child down and elevating the legs
PDA	— below left clavicle and radiates through to the back
Coarctation	— left sternal edge and between scapulae

Tricuspid regurgitation (systolic murmur) and pulmonary regurgitation and tricuspid stenosis (diastolic murmurs) are virtually never heard in paediatric exams.

On completion of auscultation, make a habit of quickly checking for hepatomegaly. In a baby, feel for the femoral pulses last as this is unpleasant and will often make a baby cry. Always offer to measure the blood pressure although you are rarely required to do this in the short cases. Use a cuff which covers at least 2/3 of the upper arm, with a bladder which completely encircles the arm. It is perfectly reasonable to assess the systolic pressure by palpation of the brachial pulse in a young child. If you cannot obtain a reliable blood pressure by palpation, do not offer to use the 'flush' method as it is very inaccurate. It would be more sensible to suggest using an automatic oscillometric device or a Doppler ultrasound probe. In an older child, you should auscultate to determine systolic and diastolic (Korotkoff phase IV) pressures. These vary with age but as a rough guide, in children:

mean diastolic = 55 + age in years
mean systolic   = 90 + age in years

Common cardiovascular long cases

Any of the cardiovascular short cases may be used as a long case but this is more likely if the condition is complex and symptomatic or has required surgery.

History

(a) At what age did the condition present?
This does not tell you whether the condition is congenital or acquired, unless the diagnosis was made antenatally, but the age and mode of presentation give some clues to the underlying defect. Congenital heart disease is far commoner than acquired disease and you will be expected to know the common associations, although most defects arise as sporadic events.

Causes of congenital heart disease

Cause	Associated heart defect
1. Chromosome abnormalities	
Trisomy 18 (Edward's syndrome)	VSD
Trisomy 21 (Down's syndrome)	Septal defects in 30%, especially AV canal defects
Trisomy 13 (Patau's syndrome)	Septal defects, PDA
XO (Turner's syndrome)	Coarctation, aortic stenosis
Cri du chat syndrome (deletion short arm 5)	VSD
2. Non-chromosomal syndromes	
Holt–Oram (autosomal dominant)	ASD, VSD
Noonan's (sporadic)	Pulmonary valve stenosis (PS)
Williams' (sporadic)	Supravalvar aortic stenosis (AS), peripheral pulmonary artery stenosis, pulmonary valve stenosis

Cause	Associated heart defect
3. Intra-uterine infection	
Rubella, especially in 1st trimester	PDA, septal defects, peripheral pulmonary artery stenosis
4. Other maternal diseases	
Diabetes	Increased incidence of all congenital defects, but especially septal hypertrophy
Systemic lupus erythematosis	Congenital heart block
5. Drugs	
Anticonvulsants during pregnancy	AS, PS and coarctation of the aorta
High alcohol intake	Septal defects

The following do not cause congenital heart disease but are inherited causes of heart disease presenting in older children:

(i) Familial hypercholesterolaemia (autosomal dominant)	Hypertension, tendon xanthoma, corneal arcus before puberty
(ii) Pompe's disease (type 2 glycogen storage disease) (autosomal dominant)	Cardiomyopathy in an infant or toddler
(iii) Mucopolysaccharidoses (autosomal recessive or sex-linked)	Storage material in valves may cause stenosis or regurgitation
(iv) Marfan's syndrome (autosomal dominant)	Aortic regurgitation, mitral vavle prolapse
(v) Ehlers—Danlos syndrome (most autosomal dominant)	Aortic dissection

But not homocystinuria!

(vi) Friedreich's ataxia (most autosomal recessive)	Cardiomyopathy in an older child with an abnormal gait

Rheumatic heart disease was formerly a major cause of valvular disease acquired in childhood but is now rare, even in immigrant children. Myocarditis and pericarditis are both uncommon and rarely leave persistent signs which could be used as exam cases.

(b) How did the condition present?
In particular, symptomatic or asymptomatic?
There are three common modes of presentation:

1. Murmur: detected when examined for some other illness or at the neonatal, six week, or preschool screening checks. The conditions most likely to present as an asymptomatic murmur are
— VSD
— ASD
— PDA
— PS
— coarctation.

2. Cyanosis: there are a large number of causes of cyanotic heart disease. However, this difficult subject can be simplified if the age of presentation is known and by recalling that the differential of cases you are likely to see in the exam all begin with the letter 'T':

Presenting in the first week of life:
— Transposition of the great vessels
— Total common mixing
        total (AV) canal defect
        truncus arteriosus
— Total pulmonary atresia, or severe stenosis (with right to left shunt via VSD)
— Tricuspid atresia (with right to left shunt via ASD)
— Tricuspid regurgitation and Ebstein's anomaly (with right to left shunt via ASD)
Presenting after the first week of life:
— Tetralogy of Fallot
— Total anomalous pulmonary venous drainage (TAPVD).

3. Heart failure: unlikely to see frank heart failure in the exam but you must know the likely causes.

Presenting in the first week of life:
— Hypoplastic left ventricle
— Coarctation of the aorta
— Critical aortic stenosis
— Truncus arteriosus
Infant:
— Large VSD
— Large PDA
— TAPVD
Any age:
— Supraventricular tachycardia (SVT)
— Myocarditis
— Cardiomyopathy

There are five other more unusual types of presentation.
4. Hypertension: the differential in children is essentially between coarctation, renal disease and neuroblastoma. May present with fits.

5. 'Funny turns':

(i) cardiac arrhythmias.

Can present as syncope (pallor) or fits (blue). Children rarely complain of palpitations. Most commonly supraventricular tachycardias. Ask about any family history (Lown–Ganong–Levene syndrome).

Prolonged QT syndrome causes ventricular tachycardia and there may also be a family history (Romano–Ward syndrome).

(ii) cerebral events.

Emboli may occur when there is a right to left shunt and polycythaemia, which also predisposes to cerebral thrombosis and cerebral abscess. May present as fits, transient ischaemic attacks, or evolving strokes.

(iii) cyanotic spells.

Classically, Fallot's with infundibular spasm. Symptoms relieved in an older child by squatting.

6. Recurrent chest infections: this suggests the underlying condition is either total anomalous pulmonary venous drainage or a condition with a large left to right shunt and therefore increased pulmonary blood flow.

7. Suspected from chest X-ray or ECG done for other purposes.

8. Subacute bacterial endocarditis in a child not previously known to have congenital heart disease.

(c) What are the current symptoms?

In the non-acute situation there are few cardiac symptoms apart from a chronic limitation of exercise tolerance. Try and quantify this and find out how much school is missed. Ask about headaches, 'funny turns' and the frequency of chest infections.

(d) Is there a family history of a condition associated with heart disease, or a history of sudden, unexplained death at a young age? (Arrhythmias, hypertrophic obstructive cardiomyopathy and hypercholesterolaemia may all be familial and undetected.)

(e) What has been the treatment?

Document the dates of any catheter studies or surgery, and try to ascertain exactly what was done. Have there been any admissions for drug therapy, suggesting previous cardiac failure or arrhythmias? Is the child still taking any drugs?

(f) Is the immunization status up to date?

This is often forgotten and is very important as measles especially can be a very serious illness in a cardiac baby. Remember, no vaccine is contra-indicated by the presence of cardiac disease.

Examination   This is dealt with fully in the previous sections of this chapter. Remember to plot the height and weight on appropriate centile charts, as failure to thrive is a common complication of cardiac disease, and always measure the blood pressure. Measure upper and lower limb blood pressures if coarctation is a possibility.

Absence of a murmur does not exclude congenital heart disease. Always look carefully at the other systems as 15% of children with congenital heart disease have another congenital abnormality. Hepatomegaly is a common sign of heart failure in children but acute heart failure is unlikely to be seen in the exam.

Investigations   You must be able to discuss the logical sequence of investigation of a child with suspected heart disease. You will infuriate examiners if your first suggestion is an echocardiogram.

(a) Arterial blood gases: all babies with central cyanosis should have a blood gas done in air to confirm this. The baby is then exposed to 100% oxygen for 10 minutes (the hyperoxic or nitrogen wash-out test) and the blood gas repeated.

— If the cyanosis is due to lung disease, the PaO_2 will rise above 15 kPa, unless the lung disease is very severe in which case signs of respiratory distress will be obvious. In contrast, severe cyanosis due to underlying congenital heart disease is not accompanied by tachypnoea unless complicated by heart failure or acidosis.
— If the cyanosis is due to transposition of the great vessels or a large right to left shunt, there is virtually no increase in PaO_2.
— If the cyanosis is due to common mixing, there is a modest rise in PaO_2.

(b) Chest X-ray: for heart size, shape and situs. Assess whether there is pulmonary oligaemia, plethora, or normal pulmonary vasculature. Look for calcification of valves or vessels, prosthetic valves, and rib-notching (coarctation).

(c) Electrocardiogram: — axis
                                    — conduction abnormalities
                                    — P wave abnormalities
                                    — evidence of hypertrophy of either ventricle.

(d) The above investigations may provide clues as to which part of the heart is abnormal, and only when they have been completed should an echocardiogram be considered. Echocardiography performed 'blind' is as difficult as physical examination without a history! The echo is an inappropriate tool for sorting out whether every murmur is innocent or not. This is usually a clinical assessment, aided by ECG and chest X-ray. Most conditions causing cyanosis in the newborn can be recognized on echo. It can also provide useful information in acyanotic disease (septal defects, duct or valvular disease), particularly if accompanied by Doppler measurements of flow velocity.

(e) Cardiac catheter: echocardiography has supplanted many of the indications for cardiac catheterization, which may be of the right or left sides. Catheterization continues to be used to measure the pressure gradient across a stenosed valve or outflow obstruction, to quantify accurately the size of a shunt, and to define the exact anatomy of complex lesions for which surgery is considered.

Treatment   You would be expected to know how to manage the following:

(a) The blue baby:
— O_2 is useless unless it has been demonstrated to improve the PaO_2.
— A prostaglandin infusion is started if the condition is 'duct dependent'.
— Know the indications and side-effects.
— Keep warm, correct acidosis and prevent hypoglycaemia.
— A dopamine infusion may correct hypotension.
— Ventilation may be necessary if there is severe heart failure or apnoeas secondary to prostaglandins.

(b) Heart failure:
— Diuretics in the first instance: a combination of a loop diuretic and a potassium sparing diuretic avoids the need for potassium supplements, which are unpalatable for an infant.
— Passage of a nasogastric tube reduces the work of feeding. High calorie feeds with diuretics should be used rather than fluid restriction as these babies often have high metabolic rates.
— The efficacy of treatment is monitored by daily weights and assessment of liver size. If the above treatment is unsuccessful, digoxin should be started (there is very rarely any need for rapid digitalization) and added inspired oxygen may be necessary.
— Surgery for the underlying condition should not be considered until there has been an adequate trial of medical therapy.

(c) Arrhythmias:
— The only common arrhythmia in general paediatric practice is supraventricular tachycardia (SVT). 25% have an underlying defect, commonly Wolf–Parkinson–White syndrome or Ebstein's anomaly. If there is evidence of heart failure, the arrhythmia has been present for some time and treatment is urgent.
— Give oxygen by mask.
— Vagal stimulation (eyeball pressure, carotid sinus massage, ice pack over the face) is always tried but is rarely effective.

Adenosine

72:1
close at 4-5
if secundum.
Earlier, 2-3 Per
problem.

— Verapamil has a high incidence of side-effects. Digoxin should be tried, but if this is ineffective or treatment is urgent, direct current, synchronous cardioversion is used.
— Many of these children will have recurrences. Parents must be told of the warning signs. Prophylaxis may be indicated for frequent or intractable attacks.
(d) Antibiotic prophylaxis of endocarditis.

(e) You would not be expected to know the intricate details of every operation for congenital heart disease but you would be expected to be able to discuss whether medical or surgical therapy was appropriate for common defects and to be familiar with current areas of debate. For example:
1. Medical or surgical treatment of a VSD large enough to cause heart failure.
2. The size of shunt which warrants closure of an ASD, and at what age.
3. Medical or surgical treatment of a PDA in a premature infant.
4. Primary switch operation versus balloon septostomy and Mustard operation for transposition of the great vessels.
5. Total correction versus a systemic to pulmonary shunt in Fallot's tetralogy.
6. Correction of AV canal defects, especially in Down's syndrome children.

Common cardiovascular short cases

There is a plethora of complex congenital heart conditions but only nine common lesions, consisting of three 'holes', three 'blocked pipes' and three 'blue babies'

Acyanotic group: these represent two-thirds of cases, are usually simple, and there is either a left to right shunt, or obstruction to flow, i.e. three 'holes'
In order most commonly seen:
1. Ventricular septal defect (VSD)
2. Atrial septal defect (ASD)
3. Patent ductus arteriosus (PDA)
All three conditions can lead to an Eisenmenger's syndrome (pulmonary hypertension and reversal of the shunt, cyanosis developing as a result) in later life if a large lesion is not detected and treated.

or three 'blocked pipes'
In order most commonly seen:
1. Pulmonary stenosis (PS)
2. Coarctation of the aorta
3. Aortic stenosis (AS)
Of course, any of these six lesions can occur in combination but they usually occur in isolation and hence are termed simple.

Cyanotic group: account for the remaining one-third of cases and are often complex lesions. By definition, there is a significant right to left shunt, or separate pulmonary and systemic circulations (transposition), but this is often complicated by other anomalies, i.e. three 'blue babies'.

In order most commonly seen:
1. Transposition of the great vessels
2. Tetralogy of Fallot
3. Pulmonary atresia

Atrial septal defect (ostium secundum)

Most are asymptomatic and present as a heart murmur.
On examination:
— pink
— normal pulses
— soft, systolic pulmonary flow murmur
— mid-diastolic tricuspid flow murmur if left to right shunt at atrial level is large
— wide (delayed closure of pulmonary valve) and fixed (the atrial communication abolishes respiratory effect) splitting of the second sound

You are less likely to see an uncorrected ostium primum defect. The child may well be symptomatic and in addition to the above signs, there may be biventricular hypertrophy and a pansystolic murmur at the apex signifying mitral regurgitation. Many children with an ostium primum defect have Down's syndrome.

Ventricular septal defect

This is the commonest congenital heart defect and a very common short case. Exam cases are more likely to have a small defect (maladie de Roger) and by asymptomatic.
On examination:
— pink
— normal pulses
— no ventricular hypertrophy or cardiomegaly but perhaps a systolic thrill at the left sternal edge
— harsh, pansystolic murmur at lower LSE which does not radiate widely
— normal 1st and 2nd sounds

With a larger and more severe defect, there is cardiomegaly due to biventricular hypertrophy, a mid-diastolic mitral flow murmur, and the pulmonary component of the second sound may be delayed and louder due to the increased right ventricular output. The assessment of severity is particularly important as it is a guide to the likelihood of spontaneous closure and the need for surgery.

Coarctation

The commonest presentations beyond the neonatal period are as headaches, hypertension or a murmur:
— pink
— absent, reduced or delayed femoral pulses
— in a minority of cases, the left radial pulse is delayed because the narrowing is proximal to the origin of the left subclavian
— right arm systolic blood pressure is elevated and exceeds

lower limb systolic by more than 20 mmHg
— clinical left ventricular hypertrophy
— a mid- or pansystolic murmur may be audible over the praecordium but more typically it is loudest between the scapulae. After auscultating at the back, deliberately palpate for collateral pulsation over the scapulae.

Aortic valve stenosis Usually, the murmur is picked up as an incidental finding. However, it should enter the differential of 'funny turns', especially exertional syncope:
— pink
— small volume, plateau pulse
— clinical left ventricular hypertrophy. A systolic thrill may also be palpable at the left sternal edge or over the aortic area or in the suprasternal notch
— ejection systolic murmur at the left sternal edge but radiating up to the aortic area and possibly into the carotids
— an ejection click may precede the murmur
— if severe stenosis, splitting of the 2nd sound is narrowed or even reversed
Could this be hypertrophic obstructive cardiomyopathy (jerky pulse and no ejection click) or Williams' syndrome (dysmorphic, mentally retarded, supravalvular aortic stenosis and stellate calcification of the iris)?

Fallot's tetralogy This combination of VSD, pulmonary stenosis, over-riding aorta and right ventricular hypertrophy may present as 'funny turns' with cyanotic attacks or loss of consciousness. Alternatively, cyanosis may be present all the time, there is shortness of breath on exertion, and squatting may relieve the dyspnoea somewhat:
— clubbing
— cyanosis and plethoric facies (can be difficult to differentiate)
— parasternal heave of right ventricular hypertrophy
— ejection systolic murmur over the pulmonary area
— single 2nd heart sound
Look for a scar and listen for a continuous murmur, indicating that a shunt procedure has been performed to bypass the pulmonary narrowing. Blalock shunt: left or right subclavian to pulmonary artery. Waterston: aorta to right pulmonary artery (rarely performed nowadays). Look out for neurological asymmetry suggesting previous stroke or cerebral abscess, two recognized complications of Fallot's tetralogy.

Patent ductus arteriosus This defect is more common if the child was born prematurely. It may just be a murmur but if the left to right shunt is large, a 'full house' may be apparent:
— pink
— full volume, collapsing pulses

— wide pulse pressure on sphygmomanometry
— apex beat is displaced (volume overload)
— harsh systolic or continuous ('machinery') murmur loudest under the left clavicle and radiating through to below the right scapula.

Pulmonary stenosis This is usually an asymptomatic murmur. There may be a history of cyanotic attacks from intermittent right to left shunting through a persistent foramen ovale:
— pink
— normal pulses
— parasternal heave of right ventricular hypertrophy
— ejection systolic murmur loudest in pulmonary area. A click may precede this but the murmur does not radiate to the carotids.
— if severe stenosis, 2nd sound splits widely (but nor fixed).

Pulmonary hypertension May complicate any lesion in which there has been increased pulmonary blood flow (i.e. 'holes' with left to right shunt), and rarely pulmonary hypertension can occur as a primary disorder (idiopathic, congenital rubella syndrome and Williams' syndrome):
— parasternal heave
— loud pulmonary 2nd sound
— in addition, there may be systolic pulmonary flow murmur or diastolic murmur of pulmonary regurgitation

If a left to right shunt causes irreversible pulmonary hypertension, this is called Eisenmenger's syndrome. This may progress until pulmonary artery pressure exceeds systemic pressure and the shunt then becomes right to left, leading to cyanosis and clubbing in addition to the other features listed above. Closure of the 'hole' should not be undertaken once this complication has occurred.

5. The respiratory system

When examining this system, the emphasis differs depending on the age of the child. The younger the child, the more important is the phase of inspection, the more difficult are palpation and percussion, and the less informative is auscultation.

Inspection It is crucial to allow a period of time to observe an infant or toddler and indeed when examining the respiratory system of a neonate, observation provides 90% of the information. Use your ears as well as your eyes. Do not undress a young child, especially a sleeping one, until you have established:

1. The respiratory rate. Never guess this or say that it is 'about 40' for example. Count the rate exactly by watching chest or abdominal movements for 10 seconds and say whether this is normal or raised.

	Normal range (per minute)
Neonate	30–60
Infant	20–40
1–3 years	20–30
Over 3	15–25

2. Whether there is cyanosis.

3. If there is flaring of the nares or visible recession (e.g. suprasternal) suggesting increased effort in inspiration.

4. If there is audible stridor (inspiration > expiration) or wheeze (expiration > inspiration) suggesting obstruction of the upper or lower airways respectively.

These four questions all become more difficult to answer unequivocally once a baby is agitated or crying, and the most likely precipitant for this is undressing the baby. However, this has to be done and the top half of the child should be exposed completely after inspection has taken place.

Inspection of the respiratory system of a child of school age follows a different pattern. Introduce yourself and explain what you are about to do whilst noting the following:
— well or ill?
— receiving added oxygen?
— thin or emaciated?
— dyspnoeic?
Observe the following in order:

| Hands | Clubbing | There is increase in curvature in both dimensions and loss of the nail-bed |

angle. Clubbing is over-diagnosed by
candidates so avoid 'early clubbing'.
— cystic fibrosis
— bronchiectasis

Face	Cyanosis	Look at the lips and ask to stick out the tongue.
Neck	Tracheal tug Suprasternal recession	Both signs of increased effort required for inspiration. Feel for cervical lymph nodes and if relevant offer to examine the throat and ears at the end of the examination. Feel if the trachea is central by gently trying to place your finger between the trachea and the sternal head of sternocleidomastoid on either side. Is this equally easy? Remember that the trachea is a very mobile structure in young children and fixed tracheal deviation is rare.

For the differential diagnosis of swellings in the neck, see
Chapters 7 and 12.

Note any coughing, stridor or audible wheeze and whether
a sputum pot has been provided (think of brochiectasis), in
which case the contents should be inspected and described.

Undress the top half of the child completely to the waist
(except for an adolescent girl). Never try to auscultate the
chest through or underneath clothing.

Observe the chest for:

Deformity	Pectus excavatum	Depressed sternum
	Pectus carinatum	Prominent sternum (Both normal variants)
	Harrison's sulcus	Retracted costal cartilages, suggesting chronic condition, either airways obstruction or left to right cardiac shunt.
	Hyperinflation	Increased antero-posterior diameter suggests asthma or emphysema. If unilateral, think of MacCleod's syndrome (unilateral emphysema) as pneumothorax and foreign body are unlikely to be exam cases.
	Rachitic rosary	Swelling of the costochondral junctions in rickets.

Absent clavicles	Craniocleidal dysostosis
Absent pectoralis	Poland's syndrome. Often accompanied by ipsilateral syndactyly of the hand.

Don't forget to look at the back of the chest for:

Scoliosis	Decide whether it is convex to right or left. At the end of the examination, ask an older child to touch his toes; a postural scoliosis will not show a rib hump. (See Ch. 11.)

Recession	Intercostal	Airways obstruction or
	Subcostal	decreased lung compliance

Scars	Sternotomy
	Thoracotomy
	Previous chest
	drains

Movement	Compare both sides.

Palpation   Again, the approach to the infant and the older child must differ. Palpation and percussion are not routine parts of the examination of the respiratory system of a baby and you will certainly appear inexperienced and clumsy if you attempt these.

Pre-school children are predominantly abdominal breathers and therefore asymmetric chest expansion is a poor guide to underlying pathology. They will employ intercostal and accessory muscles when in difficulty, but measuring chest expansion by using the hands as calipers is very crude and adds little to what inspection has told you.

With an older child, most examiners would expect you to follow the established sequence of assessing expansion, tactile vocal fremitus and percussion note, before progressing to auscultation. Begin with the front of the chest. Ask the child to sit up on the bed, lying back against a pillow with arms by the side.

1. Feel quickly for the apex beat:
— Displacement of trachea and apex to the same side implies mediastinal shift.
— Pleural effusion and pneumothorax push the mediastinum away. A small pneumothorax without a drain in a reasonably well child may be seen in the exam.
— Collapse or fibrosis of the lung pull the mediastinum towards that side.
— Displacement of the trachea alone suggests upper lobe pathology.

— Displacement of the apex alone could be due to
> Pectus excavatum
> Scoliosis (convex to the right, apex to the left)
> Cardiac enlargement (think of cor pulmonale)
> Dextrocardia (think of Kartagener's syndrome and bronchiectasis)

2. Assess expansion.

Place the fingerstips of both hands on the chest wall laterally so that the thumbs meet in the midline. Ask the child to take a deep breath in and observe which thumb moves least from the midline. This side has diminished expansion and the abnormality (effusion, pneumothorax, collapse, consolidation or fibrosis) must be on that side. Only the thumbs should move; the fingertips must be kept tightly applied to the chest wall throughout.

3. Tactile vocal fremitus.

This provides exactly the same information as vocal resonance assessed during auscultation, so do not do both. We would recommend testing vocal resonance as differences are more easily detected. To test tactile vocal fremitus, place the palm of the hand on either side of the upper chest, anteriorly, and ask the child to say '99'. Most children will happily engage in this game. Feel for a difference between right and left rather than an absolute increase or decrease.

Vibrations increased	— consolidation on that side
Vibrations reduced	— collapse on that side
	— pleural thickening on that side
Vibrations absent	— pleural effusion on that side

Percussion This is often done very badly. The main pitfalls are:

1. Not warning the child what you are about to do and terrifying him with a resounding blow to the chest. A more pleasant introduction is to say 'I am going to make you sound like a drum'.

2. It is equally bad to try and generate a very loud percussion note so that the examiners can hear it as well as you. This is unnecessary.

3. Not applying the middle finger of the left hand firmly enough to the child's chest so that the percussion note is muffled.

4. Endless tapping all over the chest without reaching any conclusion. Practise percussing only twice at each of the sites suggested for auscultation, alternating right and left, and ignore minor or inconstant differences between the two sides.

5. Failure to determine where the upper border of the liver lies.

Resonance is increased in the same conditions as cause hyperinflation (see inspection). With generalized hyperinflation or emphysema, there will be loss of cardiac dullness and downward displacement of the upper border of the liver (normally, 6th intercostal space anteriorly). Resonance is decreased over consolidation, collapse, fibrosis or pleural thickening. Resonance is absent (stony dull) over a pleural effusion.

Continue with auscultation of the front of the chest before turning to palpation and percussion of the back. This allows you to synthesize the findings from palpation, percussion and auscultation of the front and sides (upper and middle lobes) before examining the back (mostly lower lobes), and avoids the child sitting back and forwards repeatedly which is time-consuming.

Auscultation You must, of course, take your own stethoscope into the exam and this should be a paediatric model, not a neonatal or adult stethoscope. The diaphragm is better for higher frequencies and the bell for deeper sounds. Neither is perfect but it is cumbersome and time-consuming in the exam to keep swapping between them so get into the habit of using one or the other when examining children's chests. If you prefer the diaphragm, always make a show of warming it with your hand first. However, we recommend using the bell for examining the chest. It is not cold and therefore less likely to make a baby cry. Moreover, most sounds in the chest are low-pitched compared to cardiac murmurs and anyway if the bell is applied tightly to the chest wall, it behaves like a diaphragm.

Explain to a toddler that you are about to listen to his 'tummy' (he is less likely to understand 'chest') but do not ask his permission. If the child appears reluctant, demonstrating on a toy or a parent shows an understanding approach, although it may not actually get you much further. Do not give up; the doctor in a clinic must be able to appreciate chest sounds between cries and rebuffs. A dummy or bottle may settle a crying baby. As always, it is best to auscultate a baby's or toddler's chest on his parent's lap.

Listen for one or two breaths at each of six sites anteriorly in the following order:
— below right clavicle
— below left clavicle
— medial to right nipple
— medial to left nipple
— right axilla
— left axilla
Perfect the habit of deciding whether there is a difference between right and left based on only these 12 breaths. You cannot listen endlessly at the same point and you will appear indecisive if you return to an earlier site for another listen.

A 3-year-old might agree to breathing in and out through an open mouth for you but with younger children you must make the best of spontaneous breathing. Ask yourself:

— are the breath sounds normal?
— are there added sounds?
— are these in inspiration, expiration or both?

Normal breath sounds are described as vesicular and are a low-pitched rustle. They last throughout inspiration and continue into expiration without a pause. However, they are heard only early in expiration, creating the impression that inspiration (active) is longer than expiration (passive) whereas in fact the reverse is true in normal breathing.

Abnormal breath sounds

The breath sounds may be abnormal in three ways:

1. Absent or reduced breath sounds, but still vesicular, are heard over
— collapse
— fibrosis
— pneumothorax
— pleural thickening
— pleural effusion

2. Prolonged expiration, but still vesicular:
— emphysema

3. Bronchial breath sounds:
— consolidation
— just above a pleural effusion

The character of bronchial breathing can be heard by listening over the trachea. It is harsh and the inspiratory and expiratory sounds are heard for the same time with a pause between. This may not be detectable if there is tachypnoea.

'Bronchial' breathing may be heard in normal children, anteriorly, below the right clavicle and in infants, posteriorly, over the hila. These are sites where major airways approach close to the chest wall. Ignore this unless supported by other signs of consolidation.

Added breath sounds

These are conducted upper airways sounds, wheezes (rhonchi), and crackles (crepitations). Avoid the term rales. Pleural friction rubs are rare in paediatrics and even rarer in paediatric exams.

1. Conducted upper airways sounds.
It is these that make examination of the young child so difficult and lead to most false positive findings. Most infants 'gurgle' and many toddlers are 'snotty'. Mentally register those sounds which are audible even without a stethoscope as they will remain as background noise while you are auscultating. Another useful ploy is to place your stethoscope on the side of the neck after listening to the chest. If coarse, variable crackles heard in the chest are obviously louder over the neck, they are certainly conducted upper airways sounds.

2. Wheezes.
These are continuous high-pitched noises arising because of partial obstruction or narrowing of bronchi or bronchioles.

They are more commonly heard in expiration (the positive intrapleural pressure accompanying forced expiration further reduces the lumen of intrathoracic airways), which is usually prolonged, but also occur in inspiration if the obstruction is severe.

Common causes are:
— asthma
— bronchiolitis (accompanied by crepitations)

Less common is unilateral wheezing:
— foreign body

Of these, only asthma is likely to be seen in the exam.

3. Crackles.

Interrupted bubbling noises, usually most pronounced in early inspiration, which may be
- (i) fine and high pitched at the bases:
    — pulmonary oedema
    — fibrosing alveolitis
- (ii) coarse and of variable pitch due to secretions:
    — pneumonia
    — bronchiectasis

In each category, the second condition is the rarer but more likely to be seen in the exam situation. There is no point in assessing vocal resonance by auscultation if you have already tested for tactile vocal fremitus.

Having completed auscultation of the front of the chest, ask the child to sit forward and repeat the sequence of palpation, percussion and auscultation at the following sites:
— medial to left scapula
— medial to right scapula
— left midzone
— right midzone
— left base
— right base

Remember that the base of the right lung is normally higher than the left base.

While examining the chest, you must be progressively reducing the differential diagnosis because as soon as you have finished you will be asked to explain your findings. Describe the location of the abnormal signs in terms of right or left, upper, middle or lower zones, rather than in terms of lobes which you think may be involved. Nevertheless, you must know the surface markings of the lobes.

The typical signs in the five classic chest pathologies are summarized in Table 5.1. None of these is very common in the exam but they do occur frequently in clinical practice. Memorizing this framework is an essential prerequisite to discussing your findings in a short case with any confidence.

Research (Spiteri et al, *Lancet* 1, 873–875, 1988) has shown that Royal College examiners reach 50% agreement on the following signs:

Table 5.1 Physical signs in respiratory diseases

	Chest movement	Mediastinal shift	Percussion note	Vocal resonance	Breath sounds
Pleural effusion	decreased	to opposite side	stony dull	absent	absent +/− bronchial sounds above fluid level
Consolidation	decreased	none	dull	increased + whispering pectoriloquy	bronchial +/− crackles
Collapse	decreased	to same side	dull	decreased	decreased
Fibrosis	decreased	to same side	dull	increased	bronchial +/− crackles
Pneumothorax	decreased	to opposite side	resonant	decreased	decreased

— clubbing
— percussion note
— decreased breath sounds
— wheezing
but that there is only a chance level of agreement for:
— displaced trachea
— tactile vocal fremitus
— whispering pectoriloquy
We would suggest that you add a similar weighting to your findings in the examination.

Common respiratory short cases

Cyanosis

See Chapter 4 on the cardiovascular system for the definition of cyanosis and the distinction between central and peripheral cyanosis. The differential diagnosis of central cyanosis, in order of likelihood in the exam, is

1. Anatomical right to left shunt. See Chapter 4, common short cases for cyanotic congenital heart disease.

2. Ventilation/perfusion mismatch. Most candidates forget that this is the commonest cause of cyanosis due to respiratory disease and is responsible for the cyanosis in:

(i) acute
— severe asthma
— bronchiolitis
— pneumonia
(ii) chronic
— cystic fibrosis and other causes of bronchiectasis
Only the chronic cases are common in the exam.

3. Hypoventilation. Unlike the first two groups (type 1 respiratory failure; hypoxia stimulates hyperventilation so that there is normo- or even hypocapnia), a significant reduction in minute volume results in CO_2 retention in addition to arterial hypoxia (type 2 respiratory failure). Acute or chronic dysfunction of any of the components necessary for respiratory drive or mechanical movement of the thorax may result in cyanosis:

— central nervous system, e.g. acute coma
— intercostal muscle weakness, e.g. congenital myopathy
— diaphragmatic weakness, e.g. acid maltase deficiency or phrenic nerve palsy
— thoracic cage restriction, e.g. severe scoliosis
An obstructed upper airway, even very large adenoids, can cause obstructive hypoventilation at night with chronic nocturnal hypoxia. However, these children are not cyanosed by day although the combination of failure to thrive, upper airways or ENT problems, and possibly signs of pulmonary hypertension should make you consider this diagnosis in a long case.

4. Decreased inspired oxygen concentration (altitude or ventilator malfunction) and rebreathing (increased anatomical dead space) are part of the differential of cyanosis but are not for exam purposes.

5. Methaemoglobinaemia, congenital or acquired, causes a slate-blue discolouration of the skin and mucous membranes due to the presence of oxidized (rather than oxygenated) haemoglobin. The PaO_2 is normal but the saturation is low.

Therefore, a 'rationalized' approach to a cyanosed child, based on knowledge of this differential, would be:

1. End of the bed assessment.
Is the child well or ill, thriving or not? Is there a wheelchair nearby?
Is he receiving added inspired oxygen by mask?
Is it really cyanosis, or polycythaemia?
A quick glance at the face for dysmorphisms associated with congenital heart disease (see Chs 4 and 13).

2. Look at the hands.
Is he clubbed?
— congenital heart disease
— cystic fibrosis
— bronchiectasis
If the skin creases are pale, it is not polycythaemia.
Feel the brachial pulse (see Ch. 4).
If the pulses are bounding and the hands warm and sweaty, possibly with a tremor, these are signs of CO_2 retention.
Are the muscles of the upper limbs wasted, suggesting a myopathy?

3. Look at the chest.
Is he tachypnoeic?
Is there obvious deformity or asymmetry?

4. Examine the chest.
If there are no clues yet as to whether the problem is respiratory or cardiac, feel for the apex beat and auscultate the heart. If you have excluded heart disease, proceed to formal examination of the chest. Don't forget to look at the back.

Still perplexed? Now it's time to scrape the barrel. Ask the child to do a sit-up or to raise his arms above his head (tests of proximal muscle weakness). The examiner will almost certainly stop you and ask why on earth you are getting a child with Fallot's tetralogy to do exercises!

Stridor   The child is likely to be an infant or a toddler. You are much more likely to see a case of chronic stridor than acute stridor but you must know the differential diagnosis for each.

Chronic stridor   1. Congenital 'floppy' larynx (laryngomalacia). Accounts for half of all cases in the community. Present from the first few days of birth and perhaps only present intermittently, e.g. when crying. Gradually resolves spontaneously so beware of this diagnosis in a child over 1 year.

2. Subglottic stenosis. Almost invariably an 'ex-prem' but there need not necessarily be a history of prolonged ventilation. If the stenosis is more distal, there may be stridor on expiration as well. Congenital tracheal stenosis is a recognized but rare entity and tracheal stenosis may also follow repair of a tracheo-oesophageal fistula.

3. Laryngeal nerve palsies. Usually present from birth unless a complication of surgery to the neck or thorax:

(i) Lateral traction on the neck during a forceps or breech delivery.

(ii) Bilateral laryngeal nerve palsy associated with Arnold Chiari malformation.

(iii) Recurrent laryngeal nerve palsy rarely associated with a congenital heart defect in which the nerve is compressed between an enlarged atrium and the right subclavian artery or aorta.

4. Vascular ring. There may be associated:

(i) Failure to thrive due to recurrent vomiting as the oesophagus is often compressed too.

(ii) Diminished left brachial pulse or evidence of other congenital heart defects.

These four aetiologies, all present from the perinatal period, account for over 75% of cases of persistent stridor. Other rarer congenital lesions include:
— laryngeal web
— laryngeal cleft
— cavernous haemangioma
Acquired lesions are mostly benign or malignant swellings on or around the vocal cords or the mediastinum and will rarely be seen in exams.

Acute stridor   The important thing is to be able to distinguish between:
(i) viral croup (laryngo-tracheo-bronchitis)
(ii) bacterial epiglottitis
(iii) foreign body
Angioneurotic oedema (c1-esterase inhibitor deficiency; autosomal dominant), diphtheria, and hypocalcaemic tetany in an infant are all extremely rare but serious and treatable, factors which always increase the weight which examiners attach to an awareness of rare diseases.
A system for examining stridor as a short case would be:

1. Listen.
Is the stridor just inspiratory, or expiratory as well (suggests either very severe narrowing or a site in the lower trachea or main bronchus)?

2. End of the bed assessment.
Does the child look distressed, or well adapted to the airways obstruction?
Any features of DiGeorge's syndrome (branchial arch anomalies, hypocalcaemia due to hypoparathyroidism)?

Look at the head. Is there scaphocephaly (suggesting prematurity) or a large head (hydrocephaly – Arnold Chiari malformation)?

Are there any strawberry naevi in the head and neck area (subglottic haemangioma)?

3. Feel both brachial pulses.

Is there any difference between them or any sign consistent with congenital heart disease?

4. Fully expose the neck and chest.

Look at the neck. Is there any swelling or asymmetry? (See Ch. 7 for a fuller discussion of examination of swelling in the neck.)

Is there a tracheostomy scar? (May have been performed for subglottic stenosis, bilateral laryngeal nerve palsies or severe Pierre Robin syndrome. A residual tracheal scar may also be responsible for the persisting stenosis.)

Feel from behind for a goitre and auscultate over the neck for a bruit (goitre, haemangioma, congenital heart disease).

5. Look at the chest.

Sternotomy scar (mediastinal masses)?

Recession relates to the severity of the obstruction.

Harrison's sulcus indicates chronic obstruction.

Hyperinflation in an infant – think of bronchodysplasia (prolonged ventilation and subglottic stenosis).

Quickly listen to the heart to exclude obvious signs of congenital heart disease (vascular ring).

If you are asked how you would investigate chronic stridor, say in the following order:

1. Complete history and examination.

2. Postero-anterior and lateral chest X-ray and lateral neck X-ray to exclude radio-opaque foreign body or unilateral air trapping, mediastinal mass or abnormal cardiac shadow. Radiography should not be performed if the child is thought to have epiglottitis. Say that further investigation is only indicated if:

— stridor severe

— failure to thrive due to vomiting

— recurrent aspiration or choking

— associated signs of congenital heart disease

3. Barium swallow to look for evidence of a vascular ring or a mediastinal mass.

4. Indirect laryngoscopy as an outpatient in an older child; direct laryngoscopy under anaesthesia in a younger child.

Fibrosing alveolitis   The usual presentation is an older child with failure to thrive, tiredness and dyspnoea. Unlike most other chronic respiratory conditions, tachypnoea is often an early and prominent feature. Inspection may also reveal clubbing and cyanosis. Are there any features of Cushing's syndrome (iatrogenic)?

The most striking sign on auscultation is the presence of fine inspiratory crackles at the bases of both lung fields. There may also be signs of pulmonary hypertension and even cor pulmonale in advanced disease. Most childhood cases are idiopathic (also called cryptogenic and, in American texts, Hamman–Rich syndrome) fibrosing alveolitis and the only treatment options are immunosuppression, usually by cortico-steroids, and domiciliary oxygen.

Bronchiectasis
This was formerly common following measles, whooping cough, tuberculosis or pneumonia, but the incidence has declined and children seen in examinations now are likely to suffer from:

   (i) cystic fibrosis
   (ii) Kartagener's syndrome (immotile cilia syndrome):
      — cardiac and visceral situs inversus
      — chronic sinusitis
      — bronchiectasis
      — infertility in males
   (iii) inhaled foreign body
   (iv) tracheobronchomalacia

Apart from foreign body, which most commonly affects the right middle lobe, the left lower lobe has the poorest drainage and is the most vulnerable to the changes of bronchiectasis.

The dominant symptom is chronic cough (think of asthma, foreign body, bronchiectasis, tracheo-oesophageal fistula) which is usually, but not necessarily, productive. On general examination there may be failure to thrive, clubbing and cyanosis. Look at the chest for the chronic deformities of pectus carinatum, hyperinflation or Harrison's sulcus. Local-ize the apex beat.

Over the area of bronchiectasis, auscultation reveals coarse crackles but there may also be decreased breath sounds and variable wheeze confined to that area. If you have found dextrocardia and evidence of bronchiectasis, offer to examine the abdomen.

Common respiratory long cases

Chronic asthma
A definition of asthma is 'recurrent reversible small airways obstruction'. Asthma may be either:

   (i) acute and infrequent.
   (ii) episodic, with frequent acute attacks, but complete resolution between attacks.
   (iii) chronic, with persistence of some symptoms between recurrent 'acute on chronic' exacerbations.

You are most likely to see chronic asthma as a long case and therefore it is important that you make a thorough assessment of:

— the severity of the persisting symptoms
— the chronicity of symptoms between attacks
— compliance with treatment and the efficacy of such treat-ment

History   1. What is the evidence from the parents that the child has asthma? Has recurrent wheeze responding to bronchodilator treatment definitely been documented, or is the history one of persistent cough and repeated admissions with vague 'chestiness'? Perhaps there has been chronic nocturnal cough or shortness of breath on exercise without audible wheeze.

2. At what age did asthma start and were there any relevant prior respiratory illnesses, e.g. neonatal respiratory distress or bronchiolitis?

3. What precipitates the wheezing or coughing episodes? Possibilities are:
— upper respiratory tract infections
— exercise and emotion
— house dust mite
— grass pollen
— seasonal variation (spring and autumn peaks)
— animal dander (ask about pets)
Suspect environmental allergens if wheezing only occurs in particular settings, e.g. visits to the country or to a particular relative.

4. Is there other evidence of atopy (eczema or hay fever) or proven allergies (e.g. to egg protein)?

5. What measures have been taken to reduce exposure to house dust?
— synthetic bedclothes and pillows
— nylon carpet for the child's bedroom
— plastic cover for the mattress
— frequent hoovering of the bedroom
These are expensive and inconvenient changes for most families to make and the rewards may be limited. Compliance with these measures therefore suggests asthma which has been difficult to control.

6. How severe and chronic are the symptoms? Good screening questions for an older child are:
— can he keep up with other children in his class during sports?
— how many days does he miss each school term because of asthma?
— does he have a persistent, dry cough at night or wheeze every morning?
— how many inhalers/rotahaler capsules does he use a month?

7. Is there a family history of asthma or atopy? Does anyone in the household smoke?

8. What treatment is he receiving, in what dose and how often? What other treatments have been tried and failed? Does the family have a home nebuliser, again suggesting difficult asthma?

Examination   1. Is the asthma so severe or so badly controlled that there is evidence of failure to thrive? Height and weight are essential serial measurements in all asthmatics, and height can also be used as a rough guide to predict peak flows:

$$\text{average peak flow rate (litres/min)} = (5 \times \text{height in cm}) - 400$$

The third centile peak flow for a given height is 50 1/min less than the average. A low peak flow can only be interpreted if you are satisfied that the device was used properly and that the result is reproducible. This requires the child to be of school age at least.

2. Are there any signs consistent with chronic asthma?
— Harrison's sulcus
— hyperinflation (increased antero-posterior diameter, palpable liver edge)
— persistent recession or wheeze despite taking bronchodilators

3. Record pulse, presence of pulsus paradoxus, respiratory rate and temperature as the child may have come into hospital because of an acute exacerbation. If the child is connected to a 'drip' or there is a nebuliser in the room, comment on this.

Investigations   Asthma is a clinical diagnosis and investigations should be kept to a minimum.

1. Chest X-ray.
It is customary to perform a chest X-ray on first presentation. This helps exclude a foreign body and provides a baseline. Further X-rays should only be done if there is clinical suspicion of a pneumothorax. Patchy collapse/consolidation is common during an acute attack due to airways obstruction and antibiotics should be used on clinical grounds rather than based on X-ray appearances.

2. Lung function tests.
Apart from serial peak flow measurements, these have little place in the management of asthma. 99% of asthmatics have their treatment titrated against clinical response as outpatients. Occasionally, they help by demonstrating that small airways obstruction is not reversible (e.g. obliterative bronchiolitis) or that there is coexistent restrictive lung disease (e.g. cystic fibrosis or fibrosing alveolitis).

3. Arterial blood gases.
These are only useful in diagnosis and treatment of acute severe asthma when respiratory failure supervenes.

4. Skin tests.
There is little correlation between skin and bronchial reactivity and most specific allergens (e.g. cat, horse, grass) will be obvious from the history. There are many false positives and anaphylaxis is a possibility. Moreoever, the only treatment apart from avoidance is chromoglycate which is the first line prophylactic in children irrespective of skin test results.

Management As asthma is a common long case, and most candidates will have plenty of practical experience, it is difficult to excel in this case. To do well, you must be familiar with the areas which come up for discussion and be aware of the controversies in the management of asthma.

1. There are few other childhood complaints for which there is such a plethora of drugs and so many drug trials. You must be able to talk confidently about both emergency inpatient and long term outpatient management of this common condition, and most candidates obviously find the latter much more difficult. There are two aids to this:

(i) Learn the ages at which the various delivery systems can be used by children and be able to tell an examiner how you would demonstrate the use of one to a parent and child. Bear in mind that bronchodilators usually have little effect in children under 1 year.

Oral syrup	Infants and toddlers; inefficient route
'Coffee cup' method	Infants and toddlers; compliance very variable
Spacer devices	> 2 years of age
Dry powder inhaler	4–9 years
Metered dose aerosol	> 9 years of age
Home nebuliser	May be appropriate at any age if frequency/severity of attacks warrants this. Home nebulisers may be dangerous and their widespread use remains controversial. If prescribed, strict written instructions must be provided.

(ii) Understand the rôles of bronchodilator (β2-agonists and anticholinergics) and prophylaxis (inhaled chromoglycate, inhaled or oral steroids, and oral theophylline) and the indications and sequence for staged introduction of the various drugs. There is now more emphasis on early, short courses of oral corticosteroids from the primary care physician, although evaluation of short and long term side-effects of frequent courses continues. Very few asthmatics require long-term, continuous oral steroids.

A severe asthmatic may fail to achieve his potential for growth. In the context of the older child, height is a better guide than increase in weight, and drug therapy and nutrition should be geared to produce optimal height velocity.

2. You must know the 'danger' signs which warrant admission and inpatient therapy:
— Transient or absent response to two doses of nebulised β2-agonist, given 2 hours apart
— Restless (hypoxia) or drowsy (hypercapnic)

— Too breathless to talk, or chest pain (?pneumothorax)
— Cyanosis
— Absent or diminishing wheeze (worsening obstruction)
— Rising pulse rate and respiratory rate, or absence of tachypnoea (exhaustion)
— Pulsus paradoxus becoming larger
— Previous rapidly progressive attacks requiring admission to intensive care unit

3. Antibiotics should not be given routinely – viral infections are the commonest precipitant in younger children, especially in winter.

4. Despite increased awareness and improved treatment, mortality from asthma has changed little in the last two decades. Morbidity is more difficult to quantify but incidence seems to be increasing. You should be able to discuss the possible reasons for this.

Cystic fibrosis (CF)   This is the commonest fatal inherited disorder in Caucasians (1 in 2000 births) and as 50–80% of children survive to adult life, it is a disorder commonly seen in the exam.

History   1. Age of onset of symptoms and type of symptoms at presentation:
— 10% of CF infants present in the neonatal period with meconium ileus, a misnomer as there is actually mechanical obstruction rather than ileus. Ask if the mother can remember at what age meconium was first passed; 72 hours or more would definitely be noteworthy.
— CF is mostly diagnosed in infants and toddlers who present with either
    (i) recurrent cough or chest infections (50%), or
    (ii) failure to thrive despite a good intake (30%). The stools are frequent, loose and offensive.
— Toddlers present rarely with rectal prolapse.
— A few cases are not diagnosed until school age or later.
— Some cases are detected by screening in a family with an index case.
2. Ongoing symptoms:
— Frequency of admissions with chest infections and amount of school missed.
— Exercise tolerance.
— Amount of sputum production.
— Persistent abnormalities of bowel habit or stools despite treatment.
— Recurrent episodes of abdominal pain due to meconium ileus equivalent.

Other complications are:
— Sinusitis.

— There is an increased incidence of coeliac disease.

— Growth failure and delayed puberty have traditionally been thought to correlate better with the severity of respiratory disease. However, an alternative and more recent argument is that improvement in nutrition itself results in less severe respiratory disease and improved growth.

In adolescents and adults:

— diabetes (10%)

— nasal polyps (10%)

— haemoptysis (10%)

— cirrhosis (5%)

3. Take a detailed nutritional history. A component of the failure to thrive in CF is due to inadequate dietary intake as well as malabsorption.

4. Are other siblings affected and have the family had counselling about the risk in subsequent pregnancies?

5. What is the current treatment regimen?

— pancreatic supplements (what and how often)?

— postural drainage schedule

— any long term antibiotic prophylaxis?

— has the child ever received nutritional intervention (special feeds, nasogastric tube feeding, parenteral nutrition)?

6. Is the child immunized against pertussis and measles, both of which can be very serious illnesses in CF patients?

7. What has been the impact on the rest of the family of a child with a chronic debilitating disease, requiring frequent hospital attendances and admissions, and with a potentially fatal outcome?

Examination   Clinical features are very variable, both in terms of systems involved and severity.

1. General condition.

  (i) Well or ill?

  (ii) Febrile or not?

  (iii) Measurement of height and weight are essential. Most CF children are underweight despite treatment.

2. Chest.

  (i) Clubbing occurs early in CF and bears little relation to the severity of the chest disease.

  (ii) Bronchiectasis is shown by hyperinflation and coarse crepitations.

  (iii) Cyanosis, pulmonary hypertension and cor pulmonale are late signs.

3. Abdomen.

  (i) Look for scars suggesting surgery for neonatal or later bowel obstruction.

  (ii) The liver may be palpable due to true enlargement (although the liver is frequently involved, it is rarely enlarged) or downward displacement by hyperinflated lungs.

  (iii) The spleen may be palpable as a result of portal hypertension. If so, look for other associated signs of advanced cirrhosis (see Ch. 6).

(iv) Palpable masses are most likely to be faeces.

(v) Don't forget to assess the stage of puberty as this is frequently delayed in children with chronic diseases.

Investigations   1. You must be able to discuss prenatal diagnosis, both in general terms (biochemical markers, genetic markers, amniocentesis versus cordocentesis versus chorionic villus biopsy, ultrasound, which population to screen etc.) and with specific reference to CF:

— Amniotic fluid levels of a biochemical marker, e.g. alkaline phosphatase, have been used for some time to detect CF.

— In 80% of families with an affected child, prenatal diagnosis is possible from a chorionic villus sample taken at 12 weeks and using a DNA probe closely linked to the CF gene on chromosome 7.

— Unfortunately, both these methods can only be used for families with a child already affected. Carrier detection is not possible at present.

2. You must also be able to discuss confirmation of the clinical diagnosis by special tests.

— Immunoreactive trypsin (IRT) can be measured on a Guthrie type sample in the neonatal period as the sweat test is unreliable in the newborn, especially for premature infants. IRT is high in a neonate with CF but whether presymptomatic diagnosis improves prognosis is uncertain.

— The sweat test is the definitive test but false positives and negatives are common if incorrectly performed. A sweat sodium of over 60 mmol/l on two occasions is diagnostic provided more than 100 mg of sweat is obtained on each test. Other conditions associated with elevated sweat electrolytes are:

Adrenal hypoplasia
Nephrogenic diabetes insipidus
Ectodermal dysplasia
Hypothyroidism

3. A number of tests are used serially in the long term management of CF patients. You should know when to do these and what they are likely to show:

(i) Chest X-ray: indicates chronic damage (upper lobes affected first) or acute infection

— hyperinflation.

— 'honeycombing' due to the end-on appearance of dilated bronchi or cysts surrounded by thickened walls.

— 'tramlines' due to these thickened bronchial walls seen lengthways.

— in acute infections, patchy consolidation is common but abscess formation or pleural effusion are rare.

(ii) Lung function tests: show a mixed obstructive and restrictive picture. Their only value is to show the presence of any reversible airways obstruction.

(iii) Arterial blood gases: only have a place in the management of acute exacerbations leading to respiratory failure.

(iv) Sputum: sensitivities guide antibiotic therapy.
— staphylococcus aureus in younger children and permanent pseudomonas colonization in older children. Haemophilus influenzae is the other major pathogen.

(v) Faecal fat estimation: document the presence of pancreatic insufficiency and, along with serial weights, allow failure to thrive due to inadequate pancreatic supplementation to be distinguished from other causes. This test is rarely used nowadays; pancreatic supplements are simply increased until stools appear normal macroscopically.

Treatment   1. Physiotherapy: parents and older children can be taught to do postural drainage three times a day and forced expiration is also beneficial. Compliance may be a problem in adolescence but exercise should be encouraged. During acute exacerbations, physiotherapy may be as valuable as antibiotics.

2. Nebulized acetylcysteine has been claimed to loosen viscid secretions. Acetylcysteine given orally or by enema is important in the management of meconium ileus equivalent.

3. Acute infections require treatment with an antibiotic to which the organism is sensitive.

4. Regular prophylactic antibiotics are more controversial. Regular nebulized gentamicin and carbenicillin have been shown to improve lung function and reduce the frequency of admissions.

5. β2-agonists should be used to treat reversible airways obstruction. They are best given before physiotherapy and prophylaxis with inhaled chromoglycate or steroids may be necessary.

6. Pancreatic enzyme supplements are used when pancreatic insufficiency is documented. Enteric coated preparations are better as more enzyme reaches the duodenum and H2- antagonists may increase efficacy by inhibiting acid production and counteracting the bicarbonate deficiency in exocrine secretions. Optimal treatment of steatorrhoea probably reduces frequency of meconium ileus equivalent.

7. A high calorie diet is essential and fats need not be avoided with modern enzyme supplements. The calorie content of fat is more than twice that of carbohydrate. Intake of fat-soluble vitamins must be supplemented. Continuous overnight enteral feeding is advocated by some but remains controversial.

8. Psychological counselling for child and parents, especially in the teens:

— poor body image
— delayed puberty
— boys are usually infertile
— girls may have affected offspring
— terminal care

9. Combined heart-lung transplantation has been successful in a small number of CF patients, but is not a realistic option for most patients.

6. The abdomen

End of the bed assessment

Thriving or not thriving
Well or unwell
Dysmorphic or not
Nasogastric tube present
Intravenous infusion — total parenteral nutrition
Urinary catheter — spina bifida
Older child in nappies — incontinent
Afro-Caribbean — sickle cell disease
Asian or Cypriot — thalassaemia

Consider the above list whilst making friends with the child and exposing the patient from nipples to knees, unless a pubertal girl. Do not expose the genitalia of an older child.

General inspection

Hands:	Clubbing	Cystic fibrosis. Crohn's disease and ulcerative colitis but not coeliac disease. Liver disease.
	Anaemia	Look at nail beds and palmar creases suggesting malabsorption or recent gastrointestinal haemorrhage.
	Koilonychia	Iron deficiency.
	Palmar erythema	Liver failure.
Face:	Jaundice	Look at sclera. If jaundice is present, is the patient yellow or green/brown (characteristic of obstructive jaundice)?
	Spider naevi	A cutaneous vascular malformation with a central arteriole supplying a number of radiating vessels. Pressure on the central arteriole blanches the whole spider. Distributed over the area which is drained by the superior vena cava. More than three are significant.

— chronic liver disease
— Osler–Weber–Rendu syndrome
— ataxia telangiectasia

Mouth:	Observe for:	
	Pigmentation	Peutz–Jeghers syndrome.
	Ulcers	Crohn's disease.

Large tongue	There are four important causes: — hypothyroidism — Beckwith Wiedemann syndrome (look for linear fissures on ear lobe) — mucopolysaccharidoses — Pompe's glycogen storage disease In Down's syndrome, the tongue lolls forward but there is not true macroglossia.

Inspection of the abdomen

1. Abdominal distention (five F's)

Fat	
Faeces	Hirschsprung's disease. Constipation.
Flatus	Air swallowing. Malabsorption, e.g. coeliac disease. Intestinal obstruction is unlikely in an exam.
Fluid	Ascites: nephrotic syndrome is the most common cause. Look for oedema elsewhere: — pretibial — scrotal — sacral — peri-orbital — pleural effusion
Fetus	Very unlikely!

2. Obvious masses or visible organomegaly

3. Scars	Look also in renal angle for scars.
4. Caput Medusae	Veins draining away from umbilicus. If present, then look for other signs of liver failure, e.g. liver flap.
5. Ambiguous genitalia	See Chapter 7; (you should inspect the genitalia of an infant without being specifically invited to by the examiner).
6. Inguinal hernia versus hydrocoele	They can be distinguished by the following: — hernia transmits cough impulse — you can get above a hydrocoele, but not above a hernia — if it is a hydrocoele, the testis is not palpable separately from the swelling — a hydroecoele transilluminates

7. Umbilical hernia   Common in healthy Afro-Caribbean
                            Prematurity.
                            Down's syndrome.
                            Hypothyroidism.
                            Mucopolysaccharidoses.

Finally, in an infant examine the nappy for the colour and
nature of any stool and urine that may be present. After observation make some effort to warm your hands.

Palpation of the abdomen   DO NOT take your eyes off the patient's face while palpating
the abdomen (only a learner driver looks at the controls when
driving!). Gentle palpation of the whole abdomen should be
carried out initially, followed by deep palpation of all four
quadrants. Use the flat of the hand rather than digging around
with your fingertips. Examine for a liver from the right iliac
fossa. Examine for a spleen from the right iliac fossa with the
left hand splinting the lower ribcage posteriorly. If the spleen
is not definitely palpable, then lie the child on his right side
and palpate again while he is taking deep breaths. Remember
that in small babies the spleen may be felt more laterally than
in older children and a palpable spleen tip may be found in
otherwise normal neonates. Examine for the kidney on both
sides and always bimanually. There may be a pelvic kidney if
the child has had a renal transplant.
Examine for ascites if:
(a) there is hepatomegaly; (b) there are any other signs of liver
disease (clubbing, palmar erythema, spider naevi, jaundice,
prominent peri-umbilical veins); (c) the abdomen appears distended; (d) there is oedema apparent elsewhere.

To demonstrate ascites, test for shifting dullness and a fluid
thrill, involving the examiner in the latter. In the supine position free fluid, which is dull to percussion, gravitates to the
lowest part of the abdomen, and the gut which contains
resonant gas floats upwards. Percussion from the umbilicus
towards the flanks reveals a line of demarcation where the
resonance of the bowel gas becomes the dullness of the free
fluid. The position at which this occurs should be marked. If
the patient is then rolled over onto his side, the fluid moves
to the lower flank and the line of demarcation between dullness and resonance shifts.

Points to differentiate a   1. You can get 'above' a kidney but not a spleen.
spleen from a kidney on   2. The spleen enlarges downwards diagonally from left to
examination   right along the line of the ninth rib.
                              3. A splenic notch may be felt on its medial margin.
                              4. The percussion note is resonant over a kidney (gas in
                          overlying colon) but dull over the spleen.
                              5. The kidney is ballotable and palpable bimanually, the
                          spleen is not.

If the liver or spleen is felt:
— tender?
— smooth, firm or nodular edge?
— exact size? (measure in mid clavicular line)
— pulsatile? (hepatic AV malformation)
— expansile? (tricuspid regurgitation)

Percussion   If hepatomegaly is present, remember to define the upper border as well as the lower to exclude hyperinflation of the chest pushing the liver down. Specify the upper border by counting the rib spaces.

Auscultation   Listening for renal bruits is not a routine part of examining the abdomen but should be done if the child is hypertensive or has neurofibromatosis, as these are associated with renal artery stenoses. Listen for bowel sounds if the abdomen is distended or the child has a nasogastric tube. Finally, offer to examine the anus and rectum if this is relevant, e.g. in inflammatory bowel disease, but you will not be expected to do this in the exam.

Common gastrointestinal long cases

Coeliac disease

History   1. Onset of symptoms – was this related to age of weaning on to solids?

2. Know which cereals contain gluten and also that many commercially available rusks and baby foods are gluten free.

3. Nature of symptoms – diarrhoea and irritability are common whereas vomiting and constipation are rare.

4. Developmental milestones – they may have delayed motor milestones because of muscle wasting and hypotonia.

5. Change in symptoms on a gluten-free diet – often parents are most struck by the change in the child's temperament.

Examination   The child with classical coeliac disease who is anaemic with a pot belly and wasted buttocks is rare in our experience; much more likely is a miserable child with bulky stools who may be failing to thrive. However, these are physical signs which examiners tend to expect the candidate to comment upon.

Anaemia, although often difficult to pick up clinically, is commonly present in coeliac disease at presentation. An iron deficiency picture is more likely than overt megaloblastic anaemia, but red cell and serum folate levels are usually low. Look for clinical evidence of rickets (swollen wrists and costochondral joints) due to malabsorption of fat soluble vitamin D. Are recurrent aphthous ulcers present? Dermatitis herpetiformis is a well known association, and short stature and delayed puberty may be present. Of course, the patient on a gluten-free diet may have nothing abnormal to find on examination.

Investigations   Some of the investigations you should be able to discuss are:

Xylose absorption test. The one hour xylose absorption test (a standard oral 5 g dose is given followed by a blood xylose measurement after one hour) is commonly administered as a screening test for coeliac disease. However, this test fails to differentiate with certainty those patients with coeliac disease from normals. If there is a suspicion of coeliac disease then the only definitive test is a jejunal biopsy while the child is on a gluten-containing diet.

The two film barium meal. After oral barium solution two films are taken at 30 and 60 minutes and assessed for bowel calibre and the presence of thickened mucosal folds. It is very rare for the appearances to be normal in coeliac disease.

Faecal fat estimations. A laborious, unpleasant and expensive waste of time. Transient steatorrhoea is common after gastroenteritis and is present in other malabsorption states (e.g. cystic fibrosis). If the diagnosis of coeliac disease is suspected then a jejunal biopsy should be performed.

Jejunal biopsy. A normal jejunal biopsy in a patient receiving a normal gluten intake excludes coeliac disease. In the infant with chronic diarrhoea, assay of disaccharidase levels can exclude disaccharidase deficiency, giardiasis can be excluded by aspiration and examination of the jejunal juice, and a number of rare conditions which have characteristic appearances (e.g. intestinal lymphangiectasia or abetalipoproteinaemia) can be looked for. Contra-indications to jejunal biopsy include a bleeding diasthesis, intercurrent illness, and a severely debilitated infant in whom perforation of the small bowel is more likely to occur. A paediatric size capsule and experienced staff are also essential. You should be able to describe in detail how you would perform a biopsy and interpret the results.

Discussion points   1. The criteria for diagnosis, and the need for re-challenge biopsy.

2. Underlying pathophysiology.

3. Differential diagnosis of an abnormal jejunal biopsy.

4. Long term complications and their relationship to compliance with a gluten-free diet:

— benign jejuno-ileal ulceration
— non-Hodgkin's lymphoma
— carcinoma of pharynx, oesophagus, colon and rectum
— organ specific auto-immunity

5. The effect of the disease on the child and the family.

6. How and when do you approach the discussion of the long term complications of the disease with the patient?

7. What is the value of continued outpatient surveillance?

Chronic inflammatory bowel disease (CIBD)

Crohn's disease and ulcerative colitis are not uncommon long cases in the clinical exam. There are a number of important physical signs to be elicited by the candidate but success will depend largely on your ability to take a good history, gain a reasonable rapport with the patient and discuss sensibly both the practical management of the disease and of the patient and family.

History

1. Remember that Crohn's disease causes segmental transmural inflammation of the gut anywhere from the mouth to the anus, in contrast to ulcerative colitis which causes a continuous inflammatory lesion of the rectum and colon which involves the mucosal and submucosal layers only. Consequently, a history of lower bowel symptoms without symptoms suggestive of involvement higher up the intestine is more suggestive of ulcerative colitis.

2. You should be sure to determine from your history taking:

— The mode of presentation, which can be remarkably variable.
— Investigations performed and why.
— Operations performed and why.
— A full drug history with particular reference to complications which the patient may have experienced.
— Complications of the disease process. The extra-intestinal manifestations of Crohn's disease are similar to ulcerative colitis but more common. Joint, skin and particularly eye involvement should not be missed.

3. The differential diagnosis of CIBD includes a long list of infections which may cause a chronic colitis with blood and pus in the stool. In infants, cow's milk protein intolerance and Hirschsprung's disease may be complicated by a colitis while in the older child Henoch–Schönlein purpura and haemolytic uraemic syndrome should be obvious.

4. Abdominal pain, which is such a common symptom in children, is often the most important symptom in CIBD. While a full history of precipitating and relieving factors is essential, as is the site, radiation and nature of the pain, this symptom can be open to abuse by the patient who may have learnt to use 'sore tummy' as an effective means of parental manipulation!

5. A full dietary history is of some importance, not only to assess if there is an adequate calorie intake but also to ascertain if there are particular foods which may provoke exacerba-

tions. Has the child ever required a period of total parenteral nutrition?

6. How has this chronic disease, characterized as it is by exacerbations and relapses, affected the child and his family? How much school has been missed? What compromises, if any, has the family made for the child's benefit? What effect has this illness had on the other children in the family? Are there perhaps emotional and psychological problems with brothers and sisters who may resent the extra attention being lavished by friends, relations and professionals on the patient? How much insight into his condition does the child have? Clearly this will depend on the age of the child, and while it would be unwise to mention directly some of the more unpleasant complications, e.g. malignancy (ulcerative colitis), the examiners may expect you to have gleaned something about the child's own understanding of what the future has in store for him.

Examination

1. Decide if the child is in your opinion well or ill.

2. Growth data are essential; you will be provided with the necessary charts. Assessment of nutritional status is clearly important and should prompt you to measure skinfold thicknesses (if skinfold calipers are available), mid arm circumference and head circumference.

3. Carry out abdominal examination, with particular reference to tenderness, masses, scars and the perianal region.

4. Search for chronic complications of the disease process:

— mucocutaneous lesions (erythema nodosum, pyoderma gangrenosum (ulcerative colitis) and oral ulcers)
— arthritis
— conjunctivitis and iritis

5. Search for complications of drugs used to treat the condition:

— steroids
— other immunosuppressives

Investigations

1. Radiological gastrointestinal contrast examinations. Typically in Crohn's disease the mucosa is described to show a cobblestone-like pattern, the bowel wall is thickened and there may be evidence of fistula formation. In ulcerative colitis a barium enema usually shows a diffuse distal lesion confined to the rectum and colon. A barium meal may be performed to detect the presence of gastric and oesophageal varices which may develop as a complication of hepatic involvement and portal hypertension.

2. Endoscopy procedures. Colonoscopy can be performed without prior preparation or sedation on an outpatient basis. Modern flexible paediatric colonoscopes can allow a view of

the mucosal appearance of the whole of the colon often including the terminal ilium, biopsy of abnormal mucosa can be performed and polyps may be snared.

3. Acute phase reactants as a way of monitoring disease activity.

4. HLA status; there is an association between HLA-B27 and CIBD.

Discussion points   1. The approach to medical management. A balance between anti-inflammatory medication and supportive measures to maintain nutrition and avoid growth failure should be sought.

2. Indications for surgery in Crohn's disease and ulcerative colitis. Intestinal haemorrhage or perforation may require urgent surgical intervention in ulcerative colitis, but are uncommon in Crohn's disease. Growth failure and/or debilitating symptoms despite intensive and prolonged medical therapy are the usual indications for surgery in CIBD. A total colectomy may be curative in ulcerative colitis, but surgery has less to offer the patient with Crohn's disease as recurrence rates are high.

3. Annual colonoscopic examinations have been advocated by some centres for patients with ulcerative colitis to detect the development of dysplasia and therefore select those patients who require colonic resection, before the development of malignancy.

4. The management of the extra-intestinal complications of CIBD.

5. The increasing incidence of Crohn's disease, now similar to ulcerative colitis (1 in 1000).

6. Current theories regarding the pathogenesis of CIBD. The role of infection and/or a cell-mediated hypersensitivity reaction.

Common short cases   The abdomen is an integral part of the clinical short cases and, as with a developmental assessment, a candidate should expect to be asked to perform this examination. However, in our opinion this is a chance to shine. There are a limited number of physical signs to be elicited which have a limited number of possible causes.

1. Hepatomegaly, splenomegaly and hepatosplenomegaly: see Table 6.1, which is not intended to be an exhaustive list of conditions that may be met in the exam, but provides a framework within which the correct diagnosis may be sought. The candidate must know common causes of an enlarged liver and be able to search for associated signs to support his diagnosis, e.g. if you suspect right heart failure then offer to examine the cardiovascular system, or if you suspect infectious mononucleosis then ask the child for a history of a sore throat. Similarly, causes of mild, moderate and gross enlargement of

Table 6.1 Causes of hepatomegaly, *hepatosplenomegaly* and **splenomegaly**

Age group	Infection	Haematological	Metabolic/miscellaneous	Gastrointestinal	Cardiac	Malignant
Neonate	Congenital infections: *Cytomegalovirus* (++) *Rubella* (+) *Toxoplasmosis* (++)	Haemolytic disease of newborn (+)	Galactosaemia (++)	Neonatal hepatitis syndrome (+++) (including biliary atresia syndrome)	Heart failure (+++)	
Infancy and early childhood	Viral: *Cytomegalovirus* (++) *Hepatitis* (++) *Epstein–Barr* (+++) *virus* Bacterial: *Septicaemia* (+) **Sub-acute bacterial endocarditis (SBE)** (++) Protozoal: **Malaria** (++)	*Sickle cell disease* (+++) **Sickle cell disease (young child)** (++) *Thalassaemia* (+++) **Spherocytosis** (+++)	Glycogen storage disorders (+++) (usually marked hepatomegaly) *Mucopolysaccharidoses* (+++) Reye's syndrome (++) *γ-1-antitrypsin deficiency* (++)	**Portal hypertension** (+++)	Heart failure (+++)	*Leukaemia* (+) *Lymphoma* (+) Neuroblastoma
Older childhood adolescence	As above and **Malaria** (++) **Sub-acute bacterial endocarditis (SBE)** (++)	**Spherocytosis** (+++)	As above (except Reye's syndrome) and Wilson's disease (++) Juvenile chronic arthritis (++) Systemic lupus erythematosus (++)	**Portal hypertension** (+++)	Heart failure (+++)	*Leukaemia* (+) *Lymphoma* (+)

Seen in MRCP exam: (+++) commonly, (++) uncommonly, (+) rarely
Sections in: Roman type, hepatomegaly; italic type, hepatosplenomegaly; bold type, splenomegaly

the spleen should be well rehearsed and confirmatory signs looked for. It will usually be necessary to comment on the presence or absence of jaundice.

Chronic liver disease is a common short case: signs to look for should include:

— degree of jaundice (colour of skin)
— presence of portal hypertension (cardinal sign is splenomegaly)
— spider naevi (number and distribution)
— colour of stool
— evidence of pruritus
— obvious chest disease (cystic fibrosis)
— Kayser–Fleischer rings, best seen with a slit lamp and present in Wilson's disease.
— surgical scar in the region of the liver would suggest a liver biopsy in suspected cirrhosis or a Kasai procedure or modification for extrahepatic biliary atresia.

2. Enlarged kidney(s):

— unilateral enlargement; either hydronephrosis or possibly a cyst. The major differential is a Wilm's tumour which is very unlikely in the exam. Are you certain that enlargement is not bilateral?
— bilateral enlargement; polycystic kidney disease or bilateral hydronephrosis. Check the back for spina bifida, and offer to check the blood pressure.

3. Chronic renal failure: Look for evidence of peritoneal dialysis or vascular access. There may be evidence of anaemia and thrombocytopaenia (petechial rash) suggesting the diagnosis of haemolytic uraemic syndrome, or there may be evidence of a previous (failed) renal transplant. Comment on the state of hydration of the patient, looking carefully for signs of fluid overload (sacral and peri-orbital oedema, raised jugular venous pressure) and check the weight chart at the end of the bed. Offer to check the blood pressure.

4. Abdominal masses:

— chronic constipation; possibly Hirschsprung's disease
— ectopic or transplanted kidney
— Crohn's disease
— palpable bladder; look for spinal lesion
— intussusception and pyloric stenosis are unlikely
— malignancy very unlikely.

7. The endocrine system, growth and genitalia

Introduction Clinical examination of the endocrine system is largely confined to the examination of the thyroid gland and the staging of puberty. The ability to measure height correctly is important but unlikely to be required in the exam. You should be knowledgeable about and able to recognize syndromes associated with disorders of growth (e.g. Turner's syndrome and Russell–Silver syndrome, which are discussed in more detail in Ch. 13).

A detailed understanding of growth charts (both distance and velocity) is important, as is the ability to work out decimal age and calculate height velocity. A comprehensive explanation of these techniques is available on the back of the Tanner and Whitehouse growth charts.

Common long cases include diabetes mellitus, short stature and congenital adrenal hyperplasia.

Clinical examination

The thyroid

Inspection As the child sits with the chin slightly elevated, a goitre may be apparent which moves as the child swallows. A thyroidectomy scar may be present.

Palpation Examine the neck from behind the patient, palpating lightly with the fingertips of both hands. Define the upper and lower borders of the lateral lobes and comment on the consistency of the gland. Confirm that the gland, which is attached to the pretracheal fascia, moves when the child swallows some water. A thyroglossal cyst, which is fluctuant, is usually situated in the midline and moves upwards on protrusion of the tongue. Examine for retrosternal extension and tracheal deviation by palpating in the suprasternal notch. Palpate for enlarged cervical lymph glands suggestive of malignancy which is very unlikely to be present in the exam.

Auscultation The presence of a systolic bruit may accompany a diffuse toxic goitre.

A child with a goitre may be hyperthyroid, hypothyroid or euthyroid.

Pubertal staging The ability to stage puberty accurately is important in clinical practice and may be required in the long case. It is the loss of the normal harmony of puberty which implies an endocrinopathy, e.g. the presence of pubic and axillary hair in a girl without breast development, characteristic of congenital adrenal hyperplasia.

The criteria below are as described by JM Tanner (1962) *Growth at Adolescence*, Blackwells, Oxford.

Boys: genital development

Stage 1, preadolescent: testes, scrotum and penis are of about the same size and proportion as in early childhood.

Stage 2: enlargement of scrotum and testes. Skin of scrotum reddens and changes in texture. Little or no enlargement of penis at this stage.

Stage 3: enlargement of penis, which occurs at first mainly in length. Further growth of testes and scrotum.

Stage 4: Increased size of penis with growth in breadth and development of glans. Testes and scrotum larger; scrotal skin darkened.

Stage 5: genitalia adult in size and shape.

Testicular size should be recorded as testicular volume, and assessed by simultaneous comparison with an orchidometer. The testis is held in one hand and the orchidometer in the other. You would not be expected to measure testicular volume in the exam.

Girls: breast development

Stage 1: preadolescent: elevation of papilla only.

Stage 2: breast bud stage: elevation of breast and papilla as small mound. Enlargement of areolar diameter.

Stage 3: further enlargement and elevation of breast and areola, with no separation of their contours.

Stage 4: projection of areola and papilla to form a secondary mound above the level of the breast.

Stage 5: mature stage: projection of papilla only, due to recession of the areola to the general contour of the breast.

Pubic hair: both sexes

Stage 1, preadolescent: no pubic hair.

Stage 2: sparse growth of long, slightly pigmented downy hair, straight or slightly curled, chiefly at the base of the penis or along the labia.

Stage 3: considerably darker, coarser and more curled, the hair spread sparsely over the junction of the pubes.

Stage 4: the hair now adult in type, but area covered is smaller than in the adult.

Stage 5: adult in quantity and type.

Axillary hair: both sexes

Stage 1: no axillary hair.

Stage 2: scanty growth of slightly pigmented hair.

Stage 3: hair adult in quality and type.

Some facts of puberty

1. Puberty usually begins with breast development in girls and testicular enlargement in boys.

2. The mean age at onset of puberty in girls (breast stage 2) is 11.4 years and in boys (4 ml testicular volume) is 11.8 years.

3. The characteristic difference is in the timing of onset of the growth spurt which occurs early in girls, between breast stage 2 and 3, and later in boys with the acquisition of 10 ml volume testes.

4. In girls the attainment of breast stage 4 is a prerequisite for the onset of menstruation.

5. After the onset of menarche only one to two inches of growth remain.

6. Bone age is a good guide as to how much growth has passed and how much is left to come, but it cannot predict the onset of puberty or the timing of the peak of the adolescent growth spurt.

Common long cases

Congenital adrenal hyperplasia (CAH)

CAH is autosomal recessive in inheritance with more than 90% of cases due to a deficiency of the 21-hydroxylase enzyme required for cortisol biosynthesis, and 5% of cases being associated with a deficiency of the 11-β-hydroxylase enzyme. The clinical hallmark of the disease is virilization due to increased adrenocorticotrophic hormone (ACTH) causing excess adrenal androgen production. About two-thirds of patients with 21-hydroxylase deficiency are salt losers.

History

The presentation of the female child is usually with virilization of the external genitalia at birth. The degree of virilization may be pronounced such that the child may masquerade as a cryptorchid male with or without hypospadias. Inappropriate gender assignment has tragic consequences, and in the newborn baby with ambiguous genitalia this should not be attempted until the results of appropriate investigations are known.

A male infant with CAH rarely has signs of virilization, and the presentation is commonly in the second or third week of life with a salt-losing crisis. Males with CAH who are not salt losers present in childhood with signs of virilization and increased linear growth. The testes remain pre-pubertal in size indicating that the source of androgen production is adrenal not testicular.

Medical management requires glucocorticoid replacement with or without mineralocorticoid. The cortisol secretion rate is about 12 mg/m^2/day and there is 50% consistent absorption of an oral dose. You should therefore make some assessment of the patient's level of replacement therapy. Glucocorticoid therapy is usually with hydrocortisone (cortisol) or cortisone acetate in two or three divided doses with 50% of the daily dose in the morning.

Surgical management depends on the degree of virilization of the external genitalia. Cliteroplasty with reduction in the size of the enlarged clitoris is usually performed in infancy, and vaginoplasty with division of the fused labial folds if required is delayed until puberty.

A careful family history may reveal a history of previous unexplained male infant deaths.

Examination   The infant with ambiguous genitalia will usually have CAH due to 21-hydroxylase deficiency and be a genetic female. There may be isolated cliteromegaly or more pronounced virilization with partial or complete fusion of the labioscrotal folds. Other causes of virilization of a female infant include the maternal ingestion during pregnancy of virilizing drugs and, very rarely, a virilizing maternal tumour in pregnancy.

Palpable gonads are usually testes and if the karyotype is 46 XY then the commonest cause is the incomplete testicular feminization syndrome. A normal female phenotype with a 46 XY karyotype is the complete testicular feminization syndrome.

Measure the blood pressure; hypertension due to excess mineralocorticoid production is the hallmark of 11-β-hydroxylase deficiency or may be a sign of hypercortisolism. The degree of control in CAH is assessed clinically by the measurement of growth velocity and bone age; weight gain, striae and hypertension are signs of hypercortisolism.

Investigations   The commonest cause of ambiguous genitalia in the newborn infant is CAH due to 21-hydroxylase deficiency, which can be confirmed by the measurement of plasma 17-OH-progesterone and a peripheral karyotype. 17-OH-progesterone can now be measured in saliva or from paper blood spots, and serial samples can be collected at home by the patient and subsequently analysed. These intermittent daily profiles are extremely useful in the biochemical assessment of control.

Plasma renin activity should be maintained within the appropriate range for age by sufficient mineralocorticoid replacement therapy. Measurement of plasma electrolytes is unhelpful in the long term management.

Bone age estimation provides useful information about final height prognosis and degree of adrenal androgen suppression but is particularly unreliable during infancy when satisfactory control is necessary for normal growth.

Discussion points   **Prenatal diagnosis and treatment.** The measurement of 17-OH-progesterone in amniotic fluid is a reliable test for the prenatal diagnosis of 21-hydroxylase deficiency. However, this is too late to attempt to prevent virilization of a female fetus by the maternal administration of dexamethasone. Chorionic villus biopsy would allow earlier prenatal diagnosis, but current DNA probes for the 21-hydroxylase gene are not yet able to detect all patients with CAH. Some groups have treated mothers with 'at risk' pregnancies with dexamethasone from five weeks gestation until ten days before amniocentesis; if the fetus is female and the levels of 17-OH-progesterone are elevated then dexamethasone can be recommenced. The results suggest that there is a reduction in virilization of the external genitalia.

Newborn screening. The incidence of CAH is low (1 in 10 000 white births) and the measurement of 17-OH-progesterone in a filter paper blood spot is technically simple, although false positive results may occur in sick preterm infants. Routine screening would be expected to avoid problems such as salt-losing crises and inappropriate gender assignment.

Short stature   The diagnosis of the child who is short and growing slowly comprises the whole of paediatrics and is not just confined to endocrine disorders. It is possible that your long case may have a recognizable syndrome associated with short stature (e.g. Turner's syndrome or achondroplasia) or that short stature may be a complicating feature of a chronic illness (e.g. cystic fibrosis or chronic renal failure). Alternatively, the child may have an endocrine cause of growth failure (e.g. isolated growth hormone deficiency or hypothyroidism), or be short either because his parents are short (genetic short stature) or there is a delay in the onset of puberty and hence the associated growth spurt (constitutional short stature, also called CDGP — constitutional delay of growth and puberty).

We have discussed some of the commoner syndromes associated with short stature in Chapter 13, and plan here to discuss the clinical approach to the child who is short.

Information required   1. Age: Convert to decimal age to enable an accurate plot on the distance chart.

2. Measure height of child and natural parents: Plot the child's height on a distance chart. If male, plot the father's height as for 19-year-old and add 12.6 cm (or 5 in) to maternal height and plot on son's chart. For a female, plot maternal height as for 19-year-old and subtract 12.6 cm (or 5 in) from the father's height and plot on daughter's chart. The mid-parental height is halfway between the parents' centiles and represents the approximate 50th centile for the children of these parents. Establish whether the child is short for his parents.

3. Record: The birth weight and gestation. A child who suffered from prolonged intrauterine growth retardation is unlikely, despite 'catch-up' growth, to achieve his full growth potential, but nevertheless will grow at a *normal* rate.

4. Assess:
— Nutritional status by measuring weight and skinfold thickness if a pair of calipers is available.

— Pubertal status.
— Evidence of disproportion (either short legs or short trunk in relation to standing height). The best method is to measure sitting height and calculate subischial leg length (which is standing height less sitting height). Using the appropriate Tanner and Whitehouse charts, the sitting height and subischial leg length can be plotted for the patient's age and should, if there is no significant disproportion, fall on similar centiles.
— Dysmorphic or not.

In the light of the above information you should now be able to classify the child into one of the following four groups:

1. A dysmorphic child with a recognizable syndrome, e.g.
— Turner's syndrome in female
— Down's syndrome
— Noonan's syndrome
— Russell–Silver dwarf

2. Disproportionate short stature: a skeletal survey will usually be required for diagnosis.

(a) Short back and limbs, e.g.
— Spondyloepiphyseal dysplasias
— Mucopolysaccharidoses
— Metatrophic dwarfism
(b) Short limbs, e.g.
— Achondroplasia
— Hypochondroplasia
— Metaphyseal chondroplasia

3. Short but thin: search for associated chronic disease, e.g.
— Cardiovascular disease
— Respiratory (cystic fibrosis)
— Malabsorption (coeliac)
— Chronic inflammatory bowel disease
— Renal (chronic renal failure)
and consider:
— Psychosocial deprivation
— Anorexia nervosa

4. Short and fat (with increased subcutaneous fat): this would suggest an endocrine cause, e.g.
— Panhypopituitarism
— Isolated growth hormone deficiency
— Hypothyroidism
— Pseudohypoparathyroidism
— Cushing's syndrome
— Prader–Willi syndrome

The management of the cause of the short stature depends not so much on the diagnosis as on the growth velocity.

Discussion points   1. The indications for growth hormone (GH) therapy, particularly in those children who are not classically growth hormone deficient. It has been established by clinical trial that children with Turner's syndrome grow faster and taller with growth hormone and oxandrolone. Trials are underway to establish if the final height of children with genetic short stature will be increased with GH treatment.

2. The management of CDGP. This is a timing problem and the indication for medical intervention is primarily psychological. The treatment should not interfere with final height prognosis and must be safe. There is good evidence that oxandrolone (an anabolic steroid), when given in a dose of 2.5 mg daily for three months in early established puberty, will advance the growth rate of boys without detriment to final height.

Diabetes mellitus (DM)   Diabetic children are commonly available for paediatric postgraduate exams and some have become quite experienced examination subjects. The children most suitable for postgraduate examinations are often intelligent and well informed about their condition. Our advice is to establish a good rapport and *listen* to what the child is telling you.

The majority of children who become diabetic are insulin-dependent and present with a short, usually less than 6-week, history of polyuria, polydipsia and weight loss. Between 10% and 30% of children are still admitted in ketoacidosis and a comprehensive account of the management of this medical emergency is commonly required in the oral examination.

Definition   The detection of a raised blood sugar level in the presence of glycosuria and ketonuria is pathognomonic of DM. The WHO has defined blood glucose concentrations, during an oral glucose tolerance test above which DM is present. The recommended glucose load is 1.75 g/kg bodyweight (to a maximum of 75 g), the fasting whole blood venous blood sugar should not exceed 6.7 mmol/l and the two hour value should not exceed 10 mmol/l.

History   We suggest that in your clinical approach to a patient with diabetes you include the following areas. Some relevant questions are raised.

1. Presentation: A brief synopsis of the mode of presentation and any reasons for any delay in diagnosis.

2. Initial management: Was the patient ketoacidotic? How long was he in hospital? What was his initial reaction to starting injections?

3. Current management:

(a) What type and dose regimen of insulin is he on? How

does he monitor his own control? Blood, urine or both forms of testing? Who draws up and gives the injections?

(b) What dietary measures are employed? Usually some form of carbohydrate exchange system is employed with the emphasis being on a diet which is high in fibre and low in simple sugars. The provision of sufficient calories for normal growth within a framework of regular mealtimes is the goal, but in reality is often difficult to achieve.

(c) Most children will have some sort of a 'diabetic book' which they fill in, the object being to record the presence of symptoms (e.g. thirst and polyuria, or episodes of hypoglycaemia) in relation to the prevailing circumstances and treatment. A glance at the book will give you a fair idea of how well controlled the child is.

4. School history: It is clearly important to establish whether attendance or performance at school have been compromised by the condition. The requirement for daily injections may be a source of bullying and teasing.

5. Complications: It is worth trying to establish any particular areas where the child (and family) have found difficulties. Adherence to a 'diabetic diet' with regular meals and no sweets is often a problem for the child, particularly with the easy availability of 'fast' food. A common and real anxiety is nocturnal hypoglycaemia which may be on the increase as a result of the clinicians' efforts for better glycaemic control. Most parents want their child to be accepted by teachers and pupils as 'normal' but are anxious about the teachers' response to diabetic emergencies. A disproportionate share of parental attention for the diabetic child may have precipitated behavioural problems in other siblings.

6. Family history: DM occurs significantly more frequently in the parents and siblings of diabetics than in the general population. The mode of transmission is, however, far from clear.

Clinical examination

(a) Measurement of height and weight, which should be plotted on a growth chart, are essential.

(b) The search for clinical evidence of the long term complications of DM is unlikely to be rewarding in children; nevertheless, examination of the optic fundus for retinopathy should be performed and a search for evidence of a sensory neuropathy made. Postural hypotension may be indicative of an autonomic neuropathy.

(c) The presence or absence of rare but striking complications of DM should be noted, e.g. necrobiosis lipoidica, subcutaneous fat atrophy. Acute infections (particularly boils) and moniliasis are not uncommon.

(d) Test the urine. The presence of persistent proteinuria is generally agreed to herald the onset of nephropathy. Permanent microalbuminuria has been shown to predict clinical nephropathy within 10 years in insulin-dependent DM.

Psychosocial aspects: The impact of this disease on a growing and developing child should not be underestimated. Fabrication of test results and rejection of authoritarian management is common particularly at adolescence. You should gently try to establish how much insight the patient (and family) have into the condition. Do not use this as an opportunity to spell out the facts of diabetes to a newly diagnosed patient and family.

Discussion points   There are many possible avenues of discussion and because DM is common the candidate would be expected to have a broad knowledge of the subject. Some common issues are briefly outlined below.

Clinical management. Is there a requirement for regular hospital outpatient supervision, or should the condition be managed by the general practitioner at home or by specialists in the community? There is a wide range of acceptable insulin regimens, from once or twice daily injections with combination preparations to frequent injections of short-acting preparations, perhaps using the 'pen' delivery system. Flexibility is probably the key to successful management.

How reliable is the measurement of glycosylated haemoglobin in the assessment of control? The usefulness of this test may be limited by methodological difficulties in some assays, but it is a useful adjunct to spot urine and blood testing as it gives a measure of overall blood sugar control over the previous three or four weeks.

Specific complications such as the Somogyi effect should be understood. This is the presence of morning hyperglycaemia following middle of the night asymptomatic hypoglycaemia which results from the actions of counter-regulatory hormones. In this situation the urge to increase the insulin dosage should be resisted until the result of a night time blood sugar profile is known.

Future prospects for treatment. Pancreatic and islet cell transplantation have been explored in DM but, due to auto-immunity and the shortage of available islet tissue, remain experimental. Ambulatory continuous blood glucose monitoring will soon be available. The idea of a miniature portable insulin pump sited intraperitoneally which is able to respond to prevailing glucose concentrations is attractive but not yet a practicable possibility. Immunosuppressive regimens designed to curtail the process of beta cell destruction have been employed with some success after diagnosis. However, the potential renal toxicity of cyclosporin probably precludes its use at the present time.

Common short cases

Thyrotoxicosis

Graves' disease is the most common cause of thyrotoxicosis and females predominate (at least 3 : 1).

There is an increased incidence in Down's syndrome, diabetes mellitus and Addison's disease and there is commonly a family history of thyroid disease.

Examination findings:
— The hands are warm and sweaty
— Sinus tachycardia
— Restless child
— Fine tremor of the outstretched hands
— Proximal muscle weakness
— Shortened relaxation phase of deep tendon reflexes
— Exopthalmos
— Lid retracttion and/or lid lag
— Rarely external opthalmoplegia involving lateral or superior rectus muscles
— Hyperactive precordium and there may be an ejection systolic murmur
— Blood pressure is elevated, with an increased pulse pressure
— Hyperpigmentation, vitiligo and very rarely pretibial myxoedema
— Growth rate is accelerated with concomitant bone age advancement

Hypothyroidism in the presence of a goitre

The most common cause is auto-immune thyroiditis, which is more common in girls.

Examination findings:
— Cold hands and dry skin
— Bradycardia
— Reduced pulse pressure
— Constipation
— Slow speech, thought and movement
— Growth failure, as evidenced by subnormal height velocity which may antedate short stature
— Delayed relaxation reflexes
— Puberty may be delayed or advanced (see precocious puberty)

Precocious puberty

Definition: The acquisition of secondary sexual characteristics before the age of 8 years in girls and 9 years in boys. Early puberty is more common in girls but is more likely to have a pathological cause in boys. Conventionally, precocious puberty is considered to be either 'true' or 'pseudo'. (See Table 7.1.)

True precocious puberty. The appearance of secondary sexual characteristics due to premature activation of the hypothalamic–pituitary–gonadal axis (H–P–G). This may be physiological or pathological.

Pseudo-precocious puberty. The appearance of pubertal characteristics is not due to premature activation of the H–P–G axis. The source of sex hormones is the adrenal glands or gonads independent of pituitary gonadotrophin secretion. Rarely, extrapituitary gonadotrophin-secreting tumours may be the cause.

Clinical examination in girls The main differentiation is between pseudo-precocious puberty with androgenization alone, e.g.
(a) Pubic and axillary hair
(b) Clitoromegaly
and true precocious puberty with oestrogenization and androgenization (but not cliteromegaly), e.g.
(a) Breast development.
(b) Menstruation may occur
(c) Pubic and axillary hair.
The two important causes of pseudo-precocious puberty are:
— Congenital adrenal hyperplasia (21-hydroxylase deficiency)
— Virilizing adrenal tumour.
True precocious puberty is in the majority of girls (about 90%) due to idiopathic premature activation of the H–P–G axis. Other causes include:
— CNS tumours
— Hydrocephalus
— Post-meningitis
— Hypothyroidism
— Specific syndromes, e.g. neurofibromatosis (Ch. 13), tuberose sclerosis (Ch. 8) and Albright's syndrome, a triad of (a) true precocious puberty, (b) polyostotic fibrous dysplasia of bones, and (c) areas of skin pigmentation.

Clinical examination in boys If the testes are prepubertal (2 ml volume or less) the diagnosis is likely to be pseudo-precocious puberty due to extragonadal androgen secretion. In true precocious puberty the testes are of pubertal volume (greater than 2 ml) due to gonadotrophin secretion from the pituitary.
The causes of true precocious puberty are:
— CNS tumour (pineal, hypothalamic, pituitary)
— Hydrocephalus
— Post-meningitis
— Hypothyroidism
— Specific syndromes (as for girls, but excluding Albright's syndrome)
— Idiopathic premature activation of the H–P–G axis (about 50% of cases)
The two important causes of pseudo-precocious puberty in boys are the same as for girls. In addition, more commonly in boys, human chorionic gonadotrophin secreting tumours are described (hepatoblastoma and teratoma) which will cause en-

largement of the testes and androgenization from Leydig cell stimulation.

Summary of the examination of the child with early puberty

— Measure height, and assess growth rate if possible
— Accurate pubertal staging
— Palpate for a goitre and determine thyroid status
— Search for skin pigmentation or depigmentation and other signs of the neurocutaneous syndromes
— Careful examination of the central nervous system including fundoscopy and visual fields
— Abdominal palpation

Tall stature

It can be extremely difficult to recognize that a patient is tall when he is lying or sitting down. If you suspect that he is tall begin your assessment by asking him to stand, and offer to measure him and plot the height on a distance chart. The clinical diagnostic problem is to establish if the patient is tall in relation to his parents. Familial tall stature is the commonest problem in the clinic but Marfan's syndrome is more common in postgraduate exams.

Causes of tall stature:

(a) Familial
(b) Associated with dysmorphic features:
— Marfan's syndrome
— Homocystinuria
— Cerebral gigantism (Sotos syndrome)*
— Beckwith–Wiedemann syndrome*
— Klinefelter's syndrome

Table 7.1 Summary of common causes of precocious puberty

Boys	
True precocious puberty (testes >4 ml) CNS tumour	Pseudo-precocious puberty (testes <4 ml) Congenital adrenal hyperplasia (21-hydroxylase deficiency)
or Idiopathic precocious puberty (50%)	or Adrenal virilizing tumour
Girls	
True precocious puberty with oestrogenization and androgenization	Pseudo-precocious puberty with androgenization and cliteromegaly
Idiopathic precocious puberty (90%) or CNS tumour or Albright's syndrome or Neurofibromatosis	Congenital adrenal hyperplasia (21-hydroxylase deficiency) or Adrenal virilizing tumour

(c) Endocrine disorders:
— Pituitary gigantism
— Thyrotoxicosis*
— Precocious puberty*
— Adrenal disease, either congenital adrenal hyperplasia or functioning adrenal tumour*

*Final height not excessive

Marfan's syndrome

Clinical features:
1. Skeletal:
— Arachnodactyly
— Hypermobile joints
— A high arched palate
— Pectus excavatum
— Kyphosis and/or scoliosis may be present
— The span of the outstretched arms is greater than the height, and the subischial leg length (which is standing height minus sitting height) is greater than sitting height.
2. Ocular: Lens subluxation, usually upwards, is the classical defect. Myopia is common.
3. Cardiovascular: A prolapsed mitral valve is the commonest cardiovascular problem in childhood. Aortic valve incompetence, dilation of the aorta and formation of a dissecting aneurysm may develop.

Homocystinuria

This inborn error of methionine metabolism (cystathionine synthetase deficiency) has many of the somatic features of Marfan's syndrome. Homocystinuria is associated with intellectual retardation (which is unusual in Marfan's syndrome), thrombo-embolic phenomena (which may cause neurological defect), osteoporosis and subluxation, usually downwards, of the lens.

Klinefelter's syndrome

Klinefelter's syndrome affects about 1 in 500 males and is the single most common cause of male hypogonadism and infertility. The white cell karyotype reveals an extra X chromosome (XXY).
Clinical features:
— Tall and slim with disproportionately long legs
— Small penis from childhood
— Testes fail to enlarge at puberty, remaining 3–4 ml in adulthood (you are unlikely to be asked to assess testicular volume in the exam)
— Gynaecomastia may occur
Most patients have below average intelligence and tend to be immature and shy. They may present with speech and learning disorders.

Sotos syndrome (cerebral gigantism)

Clinical features:
— Birth weight and length above 90th percentile

— Excessive linear growth during the first few years which characteristically falls back
— Head circumference is proportional to length
— Intellectual retardation
— Large hands and feet
— Large ears and nose
— Clumsiness

8. The nervous system

Candidates are often confounded by a simple request to 'look at this child's eyes' or 'examine this child's legs'. To deal with these commonplace clinical tasks, you must have a well rehearsed routine for examining each part of the nervous system. The neurological examination is the most difficult of the system examinations because it consists of many separate parts and because the neurological examination, as taught to medical students, presumes that the patient is fully co-operative. Much of this formal examination of the nervous system is possible with many children of school age and above, provided your instructions are simple; this is dealt with later in this chapter. However, far more difficult is the assessment of the infant, toddler or older handicapped child, in whom co-operation is minimal and observation of what he chooses to do is more instructive than his compliance with actions which you have requested him to carry out.

It is important to understand the fundamental difference between the developmental and neurological assessments, although of course they are complementary and there will often be overlap. Developmental examination assesses the acquisition of learned skills, whereas the neurological examination assesses the integrity of the underlying nervous system and aims to make a neuroanatomical diagnosis of the site of any abnormality. Whilst the nervous system does change with age, particularly with the development of myelination, the difference between developmental and neurological examinations is best illustrated by the fact that although spina bifida and cerebral palsy may both impair walking, the vast majority of children with this delayed milestone have a completely normal nervous system.

Nervous system examination of a baby or toddler

The emphasis is partly determined by the conditions likely to be encountered in the DCH or MRCP examinations in this age group:
— Dysmorphic children
— Hydrocephalus
— Other abnormalities of the head
— Cerebral palsy
— Neural tube defects
— Hypotonia

Apart from abnormalities affecting the eyes, you are very unlikely to see cranial nerve problems in this age group and you will not be asked to test sensation.

General observation

Start with the child fully dressed and on a parent's lap.

1. Overall size and relative proportions of head/trunk/limbs.

2. Obvious dysmorphic features (see Ch. 13).

3. Posture: a consistently maintained asymmetric posture should always arouse suspicion. Look for an abnormal posture of the head (torticollis, squint or hemianopia) or the trunk (scoliosis, kyphosis, lordosis). Lumbar lordosis may be particularly obvious, and quite normal, in thin girls. A hypotonic child may sit on the lower end of the back instead of on the buttocks, while a floppy baby may show the 'frog's legs' posture when lying supine. An asymmetrical posture of the freely hanging legs may be the first sign of unilateral weakness or spasticity.

4. Movement: observe quantity and quality of both gross movements involving trunk and limbs and fine movements of face, fingers and feet.

    (i) general paucity

    (ii) asymmetrical

    (iii) accessory — tic = an identical movement repeated, i.e. a habit

            — tremor = involuntary, rhythmical alternating movement. May occur at rest or only on reaching for an object (intention tremor of cerebellar disease)

            — titubation = tremor of the head and neck

            — chorea = rapid, involuntary, irregular movements, usually of the extremities or face, which may interfere with speech or gait. The movements increase with effort or excitement. The causes in childhood, which are all rare, are:
                — anticonvulsant side-effect
                — benign hereditary chorea
                — Wilson's disease
                — juvenile onset Huntington's chorea
                — Sydenham's chorea

            — athetoid = slow, involuntary, writhing movements, usually of the proximal limbs. The commonest cause is cerebral palsy but basal ganglia disease, in particular Wilson's disease, must be excluded.

Having spent a few moments observing the overall appearance of the child, it is simply a matter of starting at the top and working downwards.

The eyes See Chapters 9 and 12 for further description of examination of the eyes. Always start the examination with the eyes because should the baby begin to cry, observation of the eyes becomes impossible. Eye to eye contact establishes rapport and it is said that a child can spot a friendly candidate by the expression in his eyes!
— Does he fixate?
— Is there spontaneous nystagmus?
— Is there ptosis or cataract?
— Are the pupils equal in size?
— Test the range of external ocular movements in the four cardinal directions by moving an interesting toy around in the child's field of view. Are the eye movements conjugate? Most children can follow an object through 180° by 4 months.

Fundoscopy and assessment of pupillary reflexes, visual fields and visual acuity should all be left until the end of the examination unless you have noted some abnormality.

Other cranial nerves Look for a facial nerve palsy. In this age group, this will almost certainly be a lower motor neurone lesion (therefore affecting the whole of one half of the face) related to birth trauma. The corner of the mouth on the intact side is pulled up during smiling or crying.

Other cranial nerve lesions are rare and difficult to test but there are a few simple clues:

1. The ability to suck and swallow in a co-ordinated and effective way is present from about 35 weeks' gestation and implies normal function of nerves vii, ix, x and xii.

2. Listen to the child's speech. Normal articulation makes lesions of viii, x and xii unlikely. Beware of diagnosing dysarthria as there are wide variations of normality in pre-school children. Dysphonia (a whispering, high-pitched voice or cry) or aphonia suggest damage to the recurrent laryngeal branch of x.

3. Symmetrical appearance and movement of the tongue requires an intact xii nerve.

If other signs deem it appropriate, you may offer to test the corneal reflex (sensory limb is v(a), motor limb is vii) or the gag reflex (sensory limb is ix, motor limb is x) but neither of these unpleasant tests should be performed routinely. Lesions of ix and x usually occur together and suggest a bulbar palsy due to a posterior fossa abnormality or a pseudobulbar palsy (upper motor neurone lesion), most frequently due to cerebral palsy.

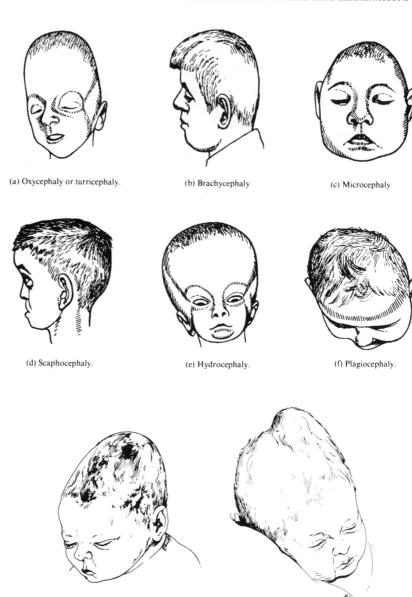

(a) Oxycephaly or turricephaly.

(b) Brachycephaly

(c) Microcephaly

(d) Scaphocephaly.

(e) Hydrocephaly.

(f) Plagiocephaly.

(g) Caput succedaneum.

(h) Cephalhaematoma.

Fig. 8.1 Head shapes (Reproduced with permission from Forfar J O, Arneil G C (eds) 1984 Textbook of paediatrics, 3rd edn. Churchill Livingstone, Edinburgh.)

The head   1. Shapes (see Fig. 8.1)
Plagiocephaly: from above the head appears as a parallelogram.
— most often a 'postural' deformity which corrects spontaneously once the child is mobile
— unilateral coronal synostosis

Scaphocephaly: the head is long in the antero-posterior diameter and narrow when viewed from the front (also called dolichocephaly).
— usually associated with prematurity
— sagittal synostosis
— sometimes Hurler's syndrome

Turricephaly: the head is tall due to compensatory upward growth (also called acrocephaly). Raised intracranial pressure is especially likely to occur with this deformity.
— bilateral coronal synostosis. Think of Apert's syndrome and Carpenter's syndrome.

Brachycephaly: the back of the head is flattened.
— Down's syndrome
— bilateral coronal synostosis

2. Sutures:
— coronal
— sagittal
— lamboid
— metopic (in the midline of the forehead due to early synostosis between the frontal bones. Cosmetic problem only.)
If premature fusion of a suture occurs, skull growth cannot occur perpendicular to that suture but continues to occur in the line of the fused suture; hence sagittal fusion results in scaphocephaly. Widely separated sutures suggest raised intracranial pressure (see below).

3. Fontanelles:
— anterior (diamond shape)
— posterior (triangular)
— third fontanelle (may be only a just perceptible widening of the sagittal suture between anterior and posterior fontanelles. A normal variant but also a clue to Down's syndrome in the newborn.)
Fontanelles usually close at around one year of age. Delayed closure (more than 18 months) suggests:
— hydrocephalus
— Down's syndrome
— hypothyroidism
Abnormally wide fontanelles at any age suggest:
— rickets
— hypothyroidism
— cranial synostosis
— rare syndromes such as Smith–Lemli–Opitz syndrome, Zellweger's syndrome and Rubinstein–Taybi syndrome.
The mean anterior fontanelle measurement (length plus width divided by two) is 2 cm at birth but the 95% confidence limits during the first year of life are 0–5 cm. In contrast to this

wide range, the posterior fontanelle is fingertip size or smaller in 97% of newborn infants.

Intracranial pressure is best assessed by appearance and palpation of the anterior fontanelle, provided the infant is sitting up and not crying. The fontanelle may be:

— bulging (elevated above the convexity of the skull)
— tense (flush with the skull but there is increased resistance to light pressure with the fingertips and pulsation at cardiac frequency is easily felt)
— normal
— sunken (implies 5–10% dehydration)

4. Head size: microcephaly and macrocephaly are discussed in the short cases at the end of the chapter. Leave measurement of occipito-frontal circumference to the end of the examination.

5. Other features to look for in the head and neck area (see Ch. 13 for general comments on dysmorphic features):
(i) Ptosis: unilateral ptosis may be due to a Horner's syndrome (pupil small) or iii nerve lesion (pupil large and paralytic squint). The most likely cause in this age group is a congenital Horner's syndrome as a result of shoulder traction at birth damaging the sympathetic chain. Bilateral ptosis is more likely to be due to a myopathy than to myasthenia in this age group. Look for other evidence of myopathic facies:
— restricted eye movements
— long, thin face
— drooping mouth
— lack of expression
Possible causes are:
— nemaline rod myopathy
— central nuclear myopathy
— congenital myotonic dystrophy
(ii) Torticollis: the head is held to one side because of:
— sternocleidomastoid 'tumour'. An ischaemic contracture of the muscle, usually due to a birth injury, causes ipsilateral lateral neck flexion and rotation of the chin to the opposite side.
— a paralytic squint; the new position of the head allows both eyes to fixate
(iii) Opisthotonus must not be confused with neck stiffness, which you are unlikely to see in an exam situation. Opisthotonus is an involuntary extension of the neck accompanied by arching of the back due to spasm of the erector spinae. Causes are:
— cerebral palsy
— acute and severe meningeal or cerebral irritation
— tetanus
Opisthotonus may be accompanied by grimacing and extensor posturing of the limbs (decerebrate posturing).

Neck stiffness is an unwillingness to flex the neck as this stretches the meninges causing pain if they are inflamed. It is an unreliable sign in infants and toddlers and is best assessed by placing a parent or toy at the outside of the child's visual field and asking him to look for it. The more conventional approach is to palpate the back of the neck with fingertips while flexing the neck. However, many normal children will resist this manoeuvre.

(iv) Carefully examine for any features suggestive of a neurocutaneous syndrome:

— ataxia telangiectasia; conjunctival telangiectasia usually appear by 5 years and later become apparent on the cheeks
— tuberous sclerosis; adenoma sebaceum is not present in the very young child but appears within the first few years
— Sturge–Weber syndrome; a port-wine stain affecting the area of one or more divisions of the trigeminal nerve, usually the ophthalmic division, is present from birth. 30% have a contralateral hemiplegia and 30% are mentally retarded.

(v) Look for the presence of a ventricular shunt.

The hands   Look for obvious fisting and quickly check for syndactyly, polydactyly, clinodactyly and abnormal palmar creases. Assessing muscle wasting in the chubby hands of babies and toddlers is very difficult. Handedness is not usually acquired until school age. Obvious hand preference in a young child requires a careful search for other evidence of hemiplegia. In children aged 6 and below, muscle tone and reflexes may be slightly more obvious on the side of the dominant hand or leg.

Textbooks often make the trite observation that much can be learned from watching a child play with a toy or scribbling, without actually telling you what exactly can be learned. Such observations tell you about:

— symmetry
— skills which have to be learned and are age dependent
— co-ordination (e.g. threading beads), which again is age dependent

Unfortunately, it may take a long time to get a young child to co-operate by playing or drawing for a stranger, time which is certainly not available in the short cases. The best compromise is to offer the child an interesting toy and observe:

— does he reach out for it?
— is there an intention tremor?
— what sort of grasp does he have?
— does he transfer between hands or indulge in mouthing?
— is there symmetry of range of movement between both hands and arms?

At this stage, undress the child down to underwear or nappy. A child still in nappies beyond the age of 3 is unusual and this is worthy of comment and may be a clue to an organic problem of sphincter control. Undressing provides much information about a baby's tone and about an older child's dexterity. Although most 3-year-olds should be able to undress with a little help, they may be reluctant in the presence of a stranger and may not want your help. While undressing the child, also look for:

— generalized wasting or specific muscle wasting
— scars of ventriculo-peritoneal or ventriculo-atrial shunts
— scoliosis
— abnormality of the lower spine

The arms   Inspection is extremely important. Look for:

1. Deformity: bony or soft tissue?

2. Muscle bulk
— Difficult to assess as toddlers have plenty of subcutaneous fat.
— Loss of bulk may be due to a lower motor neurone lesion, disuse atrophy or generalized wasting.

3. Posture:
— Shoulder adducted, elbow flexed, wrist flexed and hand clenched suggests a pyramidal tract problem (usually cerebral palsy).
— Shoulder adducted and internally rotated, elbow extended and wrist flexed (waiter's tip posture) is characteristic of upper brachial plexus lesion (Erb's palsy, usually a sequel to shoulder dystocia at birth).
— A 'claw hand' is consistent with either a lower brachial plexus or radial nerve injury, or arthrogryphosis, in which case other joints will be involved.

Only when you have obtained as much information as possible from inspection should you proceed to the remainder of the examination of the upper limbs.

4. Tone: defined as resistance to passive movement.
— A useful technique is to lightly hold both of the child's wrists in your hands and quickly shake them to and fro, watching how freely the hands 'waggle'. Again, a difference between the two sides is the clue here.
— Increased tone: is almost always spasticity rather than rigidity and reflects an upper motor neurone lesion, most frequently cerebral palsy.
— Decreased tone: may be due to a lower motor neurone lesion (spinal cord or more rarely peripheral nerve), a problem with the neuromuscular junction or the muscle, or simply due to muscle wasting in a child with severe failure to thrive. Somewhat confusingly, 'central' hypotonia may also occur in children with a higher disorder of tone control (see short cases).

5. Power:
— Impossible to test formally in this age group
— Hand preference may be due to a problem of tone, power or co-ordination and these are difficult to dissociate.
— However, a clue to power in the hand muscles is provided by the tightness with which the child will grip an object. A trick for assessing flexor power in the arms is to pull the infant up by the arms from a supine position; an infant with normal power will flex at the elbows to resist your pull.

6. Co-ordination is assessed by observing play as discussed above. Remember that co-ordination will also be impaired by poor visual acuity or squint (relatively common), cerebellar problems (ataxic cerebral palsy or posterior fossa tumour) or sensory loss (very rare).

7. Reflexes: the testing of reflexes should be omitted until the end of your examination as striking a child with a tendon hammer is not guaranteed to endear you to him. See examination of the legs.

8. Sensation: impossible to test in a young child except by demonstration of withdrawal from a painful stimulus, a technique which should never be used in exams. Good co-ordination requires normal sensation in the hands and fingers.

The trunk   A pot belly and lumbar lordosis are normal in toddlers but if either is extreme this may be due to muscle weakness. All children over 18 months should be able to get to their feet from the supine position and difficulty in doing so may be a sign of proximal weakness (Gower's sign). Children over 6 years should be able to sit up from the supine position with hands folded across the abdomen.

All children over 10 months should be able to sit unsupported and failure to do so may be due to weakness or truncal ataxia. With the child sitting and his head central, give a gentle sideways push against the child's shoulder. A normal child will keep his balance by shifting his weight to the side of the push. If the child falls sideways and has to be caught, or is dependent on his hands for lateral support, there may be an abnormality of tone or posture. Cerebellar ataxia is particularly suggested by swaying movements. With the child in the same position, catch his interest with a small toy and move it through 180°. If a child aged over 3 years cannot turn to the toy except by supporting himself on his hands or altering his seating position, truncal balance or muscle tone may be deficient.

Again examine the skin for evidence of phakomatoses (see also Ch. 13):

— Tuberose sclerosis: ash-leaf depigmentation and darker brown café au lait patches may occur anywhere on the trunk and a shagreen patch, a thickened area of skin, may be present over the lumbo-sacral area. Small fibromata are not confined to the face and particularly occur under the toe nails.

— Neurofibromatosis: café au lait patches may appear in early infancy before the manifestation of cutaneous neurofibromata and neurological signs. More than six café au lait spots, each more than 1.5 cm in diameter, are considered significant. Axillary freckling is also a feature of this condition.

Turn the child over and expose the sacrum and buttocks. Look for muscle wasting and examine for:

— Obvious neural tube defect. Is it a meningocoele or meningomyelocoele? Rarely, a meningocoele may be completely covered by skin. Define the extent of the lesion.

— If there is no obvious abnormality of the spine, quickly run your finger along the spinous processes to detect spina bifida occulta.

— Dural sinus, which is usually sacral but may be thoracic or cervical. Sacral dimples are common and a true sinus rare. Clues to distinguishing these are:

  (i) if you can see the base of the defect, it is not a sinus
  (ii) if it is low on the sacrum, in the midline, and not associated with a naevus or hairy patch, it is unlikely to be a sinus.

A tuft of hair, dimple or naevus may also overly a diastometamyelia.

— Mongolian blue spots are common over the buttocks and sacrum of all dark skinned children.

It is important to examine the back before the legs as the former may give a clue to the latter.

The legs   Follow the same sequence as for the upper limbs, starting with inspection. This is most easily accomplished by getting a toddler to walk towards a parent.

1. Gait:

— Toe walking: a normal variant in the development of some children is to walk for a time on their tip-toes. However, check that there are no contractures by demonstrating the normal range of passive dorsiflexion at the ankle.

— In-toe (pigeon toes) and out-toe (duck's feet) gaits are common, normal variants in toddlers.

— Bow legs (genu varum): again, this is normal in toddlers, but if bowing is extreme look for

  signs of rickets at the wrists and ribs
  ask about a family history, and look for blue sclerae and hypermobile joints (osteogenesis imperfecta)
  achondroplasia

Blount's disease (an acquired abnormality of the proximal tibial metaphysis) may cause unilateral bowing
— Knock-knees (genu valgum): often develop in the preschool child as his bow legs resolve and usually accompanied by flat feet (pes planus). If the valgus deformity is severe, again think of rickets and if severe pes planus occurs in isolation, look for evidence of weakness or hypermobility.
— Wide-based: normal in toddlers. Cerebellar ataxia and certain cerebral palsies cause a wide-based gait.
— Waddling: untreated bilateral congenital dislocation of the hip is rare nowadays. Pelvic girdle weakness, as in Duchenne's muscular dystrophy, may also cause a waddling gait, as may the abnormal pelvic tilt in achondroplasia and Morquio–Brailsford syndrome, both of which exhibit short stature.
— Hemiplegic gait: there is increased tone in a pyramidal distribution (hip adducted and extended, knee extended, ankle plantar flexed) so that the affected leg is held straight and moved stiffly and forward motion is achieved by circumduction, the foot scraping the floor, rather than by flexion at the hip and knee. This gives the appearance of walking on the toes of the affected side.
— Spastic diplegia: walking is achieved with the hips and knees semiflexed. Classically, if the child is crawling on his knees, the feet are held off the floor.
— Limp: describes any gait where less time is spent bearing weight on one leg than the other (see short cases).
If the gait is found to be abnormal, examine the legs for deformities, surgical scars, rashes and joint swelling and proceed to assess range of movements at ankle, knee and hip joints after enquiring about the site of any pain.

2. Deformity

3. Bulk:
— Generalized bilateral wasting in spina bifida.
— Bilateral wasting, particularly proximally, in Werdnig–Hoffmann disease.
— Unilateral wasting in hemiplegia.
— Hemihypertrophy (see short case on limping). Measure thigh and calf girth at fixed distances above and below both knees.
— Bilateral calf hypertrophy (but also weakness, hence 'pseudohypertrophy') in Duchenne's muscular dystrophy.

4. Fasciculation:
— A visible muscle twitch due to spontaneous contraction.

5. Posture:
— 'Frog's legs': the child lies with hips abducted and knees flexed. This is a sign of hypotonia, rather than weakness, in the legs (see short case 'the floppy infant').

— Scissoring: the legs cross over, particularly when the child is held supported under the arms. This is a sign of bilateral spasticity, usually adductor spasm in cerebral diplegia.
— Hemiplegic: the affected leg may be held extended in severe cases but spastic hemiplegia is often only apparent on examination and not on inspection.

6. Tone: lightly lift each leg and try to flex it at knee and hip a few times, feeling for the amount of tone you have to overcome. Alternatively, try 'flicking' the knee joints off the bed; normally, flexion will occur at the knee and the heel will remain in contact with the mattress but if spasticity is present, the whole leg is jerked into the air and remains straight. Also try to abduct each hip with the knee held flexed. It is important that the pelvis is held fixed with one hand so that movements of the pelvis do not compensate for limitation of movement at the hip.
— Increased tone in an infant's legs, even just adductor tone, is more likely to be due to cerebral palsy than a cord problem.
— Decreased tone (see short case 'the floppy infant').

7. Power: in the legs this is partly gauged from the gait. Independent walking is normally achieved between 10–18 months and the commonest causes of delay are 'bottom shuffling' and familial delay. However, walking may also be delayed by weakness, neuromuscular wasting, wasting due to failure to thrive, deformity, or mental retardation. Alternatively, walking may have developed normally and now regressed, or if the weakness is distal, the child may drag his feet. Power may also be assessed in an infant by passively flexing the legs as for examining tone and observing how hard the infant pushes against you. The ability to stand up from a lying position requires good power in both legs and in the pelvic girdle muscles. Although Gower's sign is classically a sign of Duchenne's muscular dystrophy it may be present in any child with marked proximal weakness.

8. Co-ordination: a normal gait obviously implies good co-ordination but progressively more sensitive tests are tackling stairs, running, and hopping.

9. Reflexes.
(i) Tendon reflexes:
— All the reflexes should be assessed at the end of the neurological examination. Asking a preschool child to relax looks foolish on your part and is a complete waste of time even in older children. However, talking to the child and asking him questions may distract him enough for you to sneak in that vital tap from the tendon hammer. There is little to be gained by using a smaller hammer for smaller children so just try to become proficient with the standard

hammer. Hold the hammer by the end of the handle but not as though it is a hammer!
— Biceps and triceps reflexes are elicited with the arm flexed at the elbow. It is easier to elicit the biceps jerk by placing your own thumb over the radial insertion of the biceps tendon and striking your thumb rather than the tendon directly, which is hard to find in a chubby arm.
— A supinator jerk is difficult to obtain in a young child, adds little to the information from testing the biceps, and may be painful, therefore don't bother.
— The knee jerks are most easily compared by supporting both legs with your left arm and tapping below both patellae in quick succession.
— Ankle jerks can be elicited either by putting the legs into the 'frog' position and tapping each Achilles tendon in turn, or by placing your fingertips on the ball of the foot and striking your fingers.

Root levels of reflexes are easily remembered because, in the order of testing, the levels descend from 8 to 1.

Reflex	Motor level
Triceps	C7,8
Biceps	C5,6
Supinator	C5,6
Knee	L3,4
Ankle	S1,2

An abnormally brisk reflex is usually abnormal; unfortunately, an absent reflex is not usually absent but simply not elicited. Herein lies the major problem with testing children's reflexes. Always remember that the knee jerks are the easiest to elicit and the triceps the most difficult, and interpret your findings accordingly. Reflexes are rarely absent or pathologically brisk in the absence of other signs of neurological abnormality. Do not try to elicit a reflex while the child is moving that limb.

(ii) Clonus: may be elicited at the knee or ankle if there is an upper motor neurone lesion affecting the legs. More than three beats is sustained clonus.
(iii) Primitive reflexes: These are lost, or altered, as development progresses.

2 months	Palmar grasp lost
	Stepping reflex lost

6 months	Moro reflex lost
	Asymmetric tonic neck reflex lost

12 months	Palmar grasp reflex lost
	Babinski response becomes flexor
	(down-going)

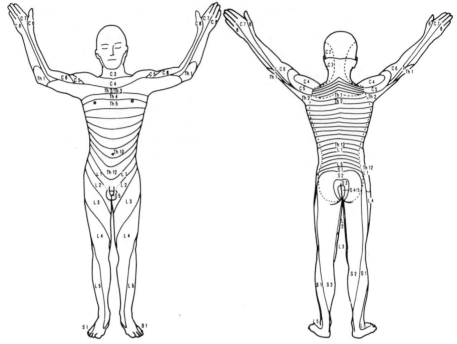

Fig. 8.2 Sensory dermatomes (Reproduced with permission from Diem K, Lentner C (eds) 1970 Geigy-Scientific Tables, 7th edn. Ciba–Geigy, Basle.)

5 years   Galant response (scratch along a paravertebral line, the spine curves in with concavity on the stimulated side) lost

Persistence of these primitive reflexes beyond these age limits reflects failure of the CNS to mature. An extensor plantar response after 1 year of age implies an upper motor neurone lesion in the pyramidal tracts of brain or cord.

Nervous system examination of the older child

Neurological cases commonly seen in the MRCP or DCH in this age group are:

Hydrocephalus
Cerebral palsy
Cerebellar signs
Children who have had meningitis or an encephalopathy with residual abnormalities
Tuberous sclerosis
Spinal cord pathologies
Neurofibromatosis
Guillain-Barré syndrome
Children who have had neurosurgery

The comments on general inspection apply as for the younger child. The essence of examining the nervous system of a co-operative child is to have a well-rehearsed system of simple commands which are unambiguous for the child and the responses to which are easy for you to interpret.

Cranial nerves
A detailed knowledge of neuroanatomy is not required for paediatric postgraduate exams and the information given here is not exhaustive. Rather, we have tried to emphasize nerve functions which can be tested at the bedside and which are important in clinical paediatric neurology. However, one useful and simple guide to the pathology underlying a cranial nerve lesion is the site of the cranial nerve nuclei.

Site	*Cranial nerve nuclei*
Midbrain	Third
	Fourth
Pons	Fifth
	Sixth
	Seventh
	Eighth
Medulla	Ninth
	Tenth
	Eleventh
	Twelfth

Olfactory nerve
Testing of smell is rarely required and should only be offered if:
— the child complains of loss of taste or smell
— the child has evidence of a visual field defect
— the child has had a frontal tumour or surgery
Ask him to shut his eyes, occlude one nostril at a time, ask him to say 'yes', if he smells anything new, and bring the test smell in from the periphery. Mint or vinegar provide strong smells and are not unpleasant for a child.

Optic nerve
You may be asked to examine any of three aspects of optic nerve integrity:
1. Visual acuity: see Chapter 9.
2. Visual fields: with a younger child, shine a light or show a toy at the periphery of the visual fields and move it around until the child's attention is caught. Eliciting the blink response from different directions is unreliable as a current of air may act as a corneal stimulus. A child of school age and normal intelligence can usually cope with testing the outer limits of the visual fields by confrontation perimetry. Sit opposite the child, your eyes at the same level as his, and explain what you would like him to do. The important point is that he fixes on your eyes and responses from the child whilst he is looking round must be ignored. 'Say yes if you see my fingers move' is the best technique as a child will lose concentration if you simply bring a small red pin in from the periphery. Test each eye separately. Test only peripheral fields

as central scotomata are rare in children (see below). The most common abnormalities in exams are:
— a homonymous hemianopia following a cerebral haemorrhage or neurosurgical procedure
— bitemporal hemianopia accompanying a pituitary tumour or craniopharyngioma

3. Fundoscopy: see Chapters 9 and 12. Ask the child to look at a toy held by his parent and explain that you are going to look in his eye. 'Whenever I come between you and the toy, just look through me as if I wasn't there'. Most children of school age are able to co-operate with this task, at least for a brief period, and it may help if the parent calls the child's name as this provides a useful aural clue as to where he should be looking. Look at the child's right eye from his right side using your own right eye and approach from 20° lateral to the point of fixation as this should bring the optic disc immediately into view. If there is an abnormality, the pupil is likely to have been dilated. The abnormalities you are most likely to see in the exam are:

(i) Optic atrophy. Only diagnose this if you are certain (see below for myopia):
— cerebral palsy
— inherited, including Leber's disease
— damage to the nerve by tumour or trauma
— following papilloedema or optic neuritis

(ii) Papilloedema. Only diagnose this if you are certain. 'Blurring of the nasal margins' and 'early papilloedema' are for the faint-hearted:
— raised intracranial pressure, including 'benign intracranial hypertension' (usually idiopathic in pubertal girls but other associations are with otitis media, steroid therapy, and abnormal plasma calcium)
— papillitis, for which the commonest childhood cause is idiopathic optic neuritis

Both of these aetiologies are associated with a central scotoma, which may be very difficult to demonstrate, and with impaired visual acuity and even blindness.

(iii) Choroidoretinitis:
- toxoplasmosis
— intrauterine rubella or cytomegalovirus

(iv) Retinitis pigmentosa:
— isolated
— Refsum's disease (deafness, ataxia, peripheral neuropathy)
— Laurence–Moon–Biedl syndrome (polydactyly, obesity, hypogonadism, mental retardation)

(v) Cherry red spot. Small red spot at the macule (lateral to optic disc) surrounded by a pale halo. This occurs in a number of the sphingolipidoses:
— Tay–Sach's disease
— Sandhoff's disease

— generalized gangliosidoses

— Niemann–Pick disease

Beware the child who wears glasses. Most will be short sighted and the myopic eye has a deep optic cup and temporal pallor. Hypermetropic discs look smaller and may have ill-defined margins but should not be confused with papilloedema.

Oculomotor nerve   The iii, iv and vi nerves control eye movements. Isolated abnormalities are rare in childhood but paralytic squints make good short cases. Look for scars of previous ophthalmic surgery or neurosurgery. Causes of palsies of these nerves are:

– cerebral palsy

– tumours

– raised intracranial pressure (false localizing sign)

– postmeningitis

– Guillain-Barré syndrome

The signs of a iii nerve palsy are:

1. A paralytic divergent squint may be obvious.

2. The affected eye deviates down and out.

3. The ipsilateral pupil may be normal or larger and unreactive, depending on the site of the lesion.

4. There is ipsilateral ptosis.

5. Demonstrate diplopia, using a pen, except lateral gaze to the side of the lesion.

Trochlear nerve   The signs of a iv nerve palsy are:

1. Compensatory torticollis.

2. A squint is not obvious. Test by asking the child to look down while the affected eye is adducted.

3. Diplopia occurs on attempted down gaze, causing problems in going down stairs, for example.

Trigeminal nerve   1. Motor division: ask the child to open his mouth and to keep it open while you push against his chin. In unilateral lower motor neurone lesions, the jaw deviates towards the weak side. A younger child may not co-operate but if he can bite on a wooden spatula and resist your attempts to remove it, power is probably intact. The bulk of the masseters may be increased in Duchenne's muscular dystrophy.

2. Sensory divisions: there are three, the ophthalmic, maxillary and mandibular divisions. It is necessary only to test light touch and this can quickly be done by asking the child to shut his eyes and to say 'yes' as soon as he feels anything, while you lightly touch (not rub or drag) either side of his face with a wisp of cotton wool, above the eyes, on the cheeks, and either side of the chin.

Abducens nerve   See above for comments regarding the oculomotor nerve. The signs of a vi nerve palsy are:

1. Convergent squint as the affected eye deviates inwards.

2. Compensatory torticollis.

3. Failure of lateral gaze to the affected side.

Facial nerve   1. The motor division: supplies the muscles of facial expression of the whole of the face. A unilateral lesion may be immediately apparent from asymmetry of the face, with loss of the naso-labial fold, drooping of the corner of the mouth and drooling on the affected side. If no asymmetry is obvious, test by asking the child to raise his eyebrows, squeeze his eyes tight shut (remember, the oculomotor and sympathetic nerves supply the muscles which open the eyes; the facial nerve supplies the muscles which close the eyes) and by making him smile.

Great confusion often surrounds facial nerve lesions but it is really quite simple. If it is a lower motor neurone lesion (i.e. anywhere along the facial nerve itself and including the facial nerve nucleus in the brainstem), then the whole of the ipsilateral side of the face is weak. If it is an upper motor neurone lesion (tumour or vascular accident affecting the motor cortex), the contralateral side of the face is weak below the eyes but the forehead muscles are normal as these receive a bilateral innervation.

2. The sensory division: supplies taste sensation to the anterior two-thirds of the tongue. This is rarely required to be tested.

3. Parasympathetic division: supplies the lacrimal gland. Inability to produce tears is a feature of some of the congenital sensory neuropathies.

Corneal reflex: This should not be tested in a conscious child as it is unpleasant and the above tests make it unnecessary. Sensation from the cornea is carried in the ophthalmic division of the trigeminal nerve and the motor side of the reflex is via both facial nerves to cause bilateral blinking.

An isolated facial nerve palsy of unknown cause is called a Bell's palsy and is the commonest presentation of a cranial nerve lesion in childhood. A lower motor neurone paralysis develops over a few hours, the eye on the affected side cannot be closed and the mouth may be drawn to the opposite side (giving the impression of spasm on the normal side). There may be a sensation of numbness but sensory testing is always normal. Over 90% of children make a complete recovery but this may take up to 3 months. Offer to examine the ears as, rarely, a facial nerve palsy is due to herpes zoster affecting the geniculate ganglion and bullae may be present on the tympanic membrane.

Auditory nerve   This runs alongside the facial nerve in the internal auditory meatus and both enter the brainstem at the cerebello-pontine angle. Both may therefore be affected by a posterior fossa tumour or an accoustic neuroma.

1. Cochlear division: conveys auditory impulses from the inner ear. Before testing hearing, always examine both external auditory meati for local disease, wax, grommets and damage to the ear drum. Is the child's speech normal? For a description of how to test hearing at different ages, see Chapter 9. If you decide that hearing is impaired, you must try and distinguish whether there is sensorineural (perceptive) deafness or conductive deafness.

Sensorineural deafness	*Conductive deafness*
Cochlear, nerve, brainstem or auditory cortex disease	Foreign body or middle ear disease
Rare	Common
Often severe	Usually mild
High tones lost first	Low tones lost first
Often congenital and permanent	Usually acquired and transient
May be a family history of deafness	

(i) Weber's test: place a 512 Hz tuning fork on the centre of the child's skull and ask him whether it is louder in one ear than the other.
— Conductive deafness: louder on the diseased side
— Perceptive deafness: louder on the healthy side
Most children of school age can perform this test reproducibly.

(ii) Rinne's test: more difficult for a child. Place the tuning fork by the child's ear and then place the base of the ringing tuning fork on the mastoid process behind the ear. Ask him which sounds louder.
— Conductive deafness: bone louder
— Perceptive deafness or normal hearing: air louder

(iii) Causes of deafness:

    Conductive deafness
    Chronic secretory otitis media (glue ear).
    Perceptive deafness

    Prenatal (60%) — inherited (50%): may be isolated or part of a syndrome, e.g. Pendred's syndrome (autosomal recessive)   Waardenburg's syndrome (autosomal dominant) Oto–palato–digital syndrome (X-linked)

                  — intra-uterine infection (toxoplasma, rubella, cytomegalovirus, syphilis)

                  — congenital malformations of the ear

    Perinatal (10%) — birth asphyxia
                  — kernicterus
                  — aminoglycosides

Postnatal (30%) — meningitis
                 — encephalitis
                 — trauma
                 — ototoxic drugs

Therefore, consider deafness in any of the following groups of children (see also Ch. 9):

Family history of deafness
Low birth weight
Cleft palate
Cerebral palsy
Delayed language milestones
History of recurrent ear infections or central nervous system infection
The parents are concerned that the child is deaf

2. Vestibular division: conveys postural sensation from the labyrinth of the inner ear. It is therefore tested along with cerebellar function in the assessment of balance and gait (see previous section). Damage to the vestibular nerve or nucleus may also produce nystagmus: involuntary, rhythmical eye movements which may be horizontal, vertical or rotary. The speed of the movements is usually quicker in one direction than the other, the quicker movement defining the direction of nystagmus. To examine for nystagmus, ask the child to look straight ahead and observe whether the eyes remain steady. Then ask him to follow your finger in the four cardinal directions and observe the direction of any nystagmus and which direction of gaze precipitates it. A few beats of nystagmus at the extremes of gaze are normal. Always offer to examine hearing, cerebellar function and the ocular fundi as nystagmus may be due to:

(i) Vestibular nystagmus: the fast phase is away from the side of the lesion and the nystagmus is worse on looking away from the side of the lesion.

(ii) Cerebellar nystagmus: horizontal nystagmus towards the side of the lesion and exacerbated by looking to that side.

(iii) Brainstem nystagmus: usually due to a posterior fossa tumour and suggested by vertical nystagmus, nystagmus affecting only one eye (the abducting eye, 'ataxic nystagmus'), or nystagmus induced by only certain movements of the head.

(iv) Ocular nystagmus: due to poor macular vision which impairs retinal fixation. This is often rotary on central fixation of the eyes and may be pendular (swings of eye movement are the same in both directions). Ocular nystagmus is frequently congenital. Remember that optokinetic nystagmus can be induced in normal children (Catford drum or a car passing fence poles).

(v) Ocular muscle weakness: often overlooked as a cause of nystagmus which occurs when the eye is moved by the weakened muscle.

(vi) 'Congenital' nystagmus: rapid rhythmic eye movements with normal vision. The cause is unknown and is sometimes familial. The rest of the examination is normal and the condition may improve with age.

Glossopharyngeal nerve   Supplies sensation from the nasopharynx and soft palate and taste from the posterior third of the tongue.

Vagus nerve   Motor fibres supply the voluntary muscles of the pharynx and larynx whilst the parasympathetic fibres supply the heart, lungs and abdominal viscera. The ninth and tenth nerves are usually considered together as they exit the skull together, run a similar course, and both are usually involved in a single lesion. They also share a common and crude test of integrity, the 'gag' reflex. Sensation is provided by the ninth nerve and the gag response by the tenth nerve. This reflex should not be elicited in a conscious child. Dysarthria, nasal speech and difficulty in swallowing are other clues to dysfunction of these nerves.

Apart from damage to the recurrent laryngeal branch of the vagus nerve (see Ch. 5), isolated lesions of the ninth and tenth nerves are rare but both may be damaged in posterior fossa tumours, basal meningitis, syringobulbia and fractures to the base of the skull. Unilateral lesions cause the palatal arch on the affected side to droop, and it does not elevate when the child says 'ah'. Asymmetry of the movements of the palatal arches may persist for months after tonsillectomy but speech and swallowing are unaffected.

Spinal accessory nerve   Innervates the trapezius and sternocleidomastoid muscles. Function is easily tested by asking the child to:
(i) Shrug his shoulders
(ii) Turn his head to one side, place your hand on the medial side of his jaw, and ask him to push against you. This tests the sternocleidomastoid on the opposite side to which his head is turned. A younger child may not co-operate but will obligingly turn to a toy or to his mother's voice.

Hypoglossal nerve   Supplies the muscles of the tongue. First inspect the tongue lying at rest in the floor of the mouth for spontaneous fasciculation, a sign of lower motor neurone disease, sometimes apparent in children with one of the spinal muscular atrophies. (A word of warning: perfectly healthy children find it impossible to hold their tongue absolutely still so make sure you look at a few 'normals'.) Now ask him to stick out his tongue. A unilateral lesion causes ipsilateral atropy and deviation of the tongue to the affected side. Do not mistake an apparent deviation of the tongue, due to the mouth being twisted as in a facial nerve palsy, for a real deviation.

Upper motor neurone lesions of the hypoglossal nerve (small spastic tongue) are extremely rare in childhood.

Peripheral nervous system

The arms   1. Inspection.

Undress the child to the waist. Look for wasting, fasciculation or involuntary movements. The best position for observing involuntary movements is to ask the child to stand with his arm outstretched, fingers as wide apart as possible and tongue out. Wasting tends to be more marked proximally in muscular dystrophies and myopathies and more marked distally in neuropathies. There may be simultaneous wasting and pseudohypertrophy of different muscle groups in Duchenne's muscular dystrophy.

'Which hand do you write with?' 'Stretch out your arms and play the piano', demonstrating the action yourself. This will give you an idea of any gross asymmetry between the upper limbs before you begin more detailed assessment. If there is obvious asymmetry, always examine the normal side first.

2. Assess tone.

'Would it hurt if I were to move your arm?'. Passively flex and extend the eblow and the wrist; spasticity is easier to detect than decreased tone. Children find it very difficult to relax but you can 'fool' them by rapid pronation/supination at the wrist or by asking them what they had for breakfast while you are assessing tone! Increased range of movement about joints is a frequent adjunct to hypotonia but do not confuse these two signs. Repeat with the opposite arm.

3. Assess power.

Many candidates end up confusing the child and themselves when they attempt to test the child's power. The crucial points are:

    (i)   have a simple system rather than an exhaustive one
    (ii) first demonstrate what action you want the child to make, using your own hand or arm
   (iii) put the child's arm in the position you want to test and then get him to push against you

Place the child's arm so that they are about 45° away from his body.

C5   'Push your elbows away from your body' (shoulder abduction)

C6, 7, 8 'Press your elbows into your body' (shoulder adduction)

Bend his arm so that the elbow is a right angle.

C5, 6 'Pull me towards you' (elbow flexion)

C7, 8 'Now try and straighten your arm' (elbow extension)

Ask him to make a fist.

C6, 7 'Don't let me bend your wrist' Try to extend and flex the wrist by pushing against the child.

T1 'Spread your fingers. Don't let me squeeze them together'.

This simple screen will detect most causes of weakness in the upper limbs. More detailed testing will result in loss of concentration both by the child and the examiners and is not worthwhile as isolated muscle and peripheral nerve lesions are rare in childhood.

Power may be graded:

0	No contraction
1	Flicker of contraction
2	Active movement, with gravity eliminated (often difficult to test)
3	Active movement against gravity
4	Movement against resistance
5	Normal power

However, you are only likely to be expected to say whether power is normal, reduced or absent.

4. Reflexes.

Test these as described for younger children. Reflexes are either absent, normal or increased; some children have quite brisk reflexes but if there are no other signs of upper motor neurone weakness, assume the reflexes are normal. If you cannot elicit the reflexes but there are no other signs of lower motor neurone or muscle weakness, try Jendrassik's manoeuvre. Demonstrate to the child that you want him to screw up his face (or to pull his hands against each other if testing reflexes in the legs) on your command. The crucial point is that you must get him to do this just before you strike the tendon, otherwise the reinforcing effect will be lost.

5. Co-ordination.

This is a composite function requiring normal motor, sensory and cerebellar systems and there is a very wide range among normal children. Again, therefore, do not make too much of these tests unless supported by other abnormal signs. Tests of co-ordination are:

(i) Finger to nose touching.

'Touch your nose and then my finger and keep going until I say stop.' You may actually have to take hold of the child's finger and show him what to do a few times. The test has not been performed correctly unless the movements are executed fairly quickly and you move your finger around in the field of vision (this test of co-ordination also requires normal vision) to provide a different target each time. You are looking for intention tremor (the child's hand oscillates as it approaches the taget) and past pointing (he overshoots or simply misses the target), both signs of cerebellar disease.

(ii) Dysdiadochokinesia.

Show the child that you want him to tap one hand with the other, alternately tapping with the palm and back of the hand. Other examples of rapidly alternating actions are to mimic piano playing and to touch the fingers of the hand alternately with the thumb of the same hand. Children are always markedly better at these sort of tasks with their dominant hand and you must allow for this. Slowness and clumsiness at such tasks are classically attributed to cerebellar disease but we must emphasize that abnormalities of tone or power in that limb will produce similar difficulties. Diadochokinesia should be smooth and rapid by the age of 8 years.

(iii) Writing and drawing.

These activities require enormous efforts of co-ordination, of course, but as you will not have a baseline for that child, as there is such wide variation with age and ability, and as they take too long for the short cases, we would not advise using these as tests of co-ordination.

6.   Sensation (Fig. 8.2, p. 92).

You are unlikely to be asked to test sensation in a short case but you would be expected to do this for a neurological long case. Do not test for pain or temperature sensation unless you are considering syringomyelia (lower motor neurone weakness in the arms, spasticity in the legs, possibly an associated spina bifida or sacral naevus) in which case there is loss of pain and temperature sensation in a cape distribution with light touch and proprioception unaffected ('dissociated sensory loss').

(i) Light touch.

Use a wisp of cotton wool and demonstrate the sensation this will cause. Ask the child to close his eyes and to say 'yes' immediately he feels you touch him. Touch the skin lightly at each of the following sites; do not rub the cotton wool along the skin.

Lateral surface upper arm	C5
Tip of thumb	C6
Web between index and middle fingers	C7
Tip of little finger	C8
Medial surface lower arm	T1
Medial surface upper arm	T2

This simple method of sensory testing, in which the child is only expected to say 'yes' if touched, avoids some of the subjectivity and poor reproducibility for which testing sensation in children is notorious. There should be no delay in the child's response and only accept an unequivocal 'yes'. If, from previous examination, you expect there to be a sensory loss, always start from the area you expect to be numb and work towards the area of normal sensation.

(ii) Proprioception.

Children enjoy this game. Hold the middle phalanx of the child's index finger and flex and extend the distal phalanx, telling him which direction you mean by up and down. Now ask him to close his eyes and say 'up' or 'down' when you move his finger. Remember to hold the distal phalanx by the sides, not the pulp, and not to follow any regular pattern. Start with fairly large excursions to convince yourself that he has grasped the idea and then gradually reduce the size of the movement. Remember that normal proprioception is very sensitive and a normal child will detect movements of only a few millimetres. Try it out! It is worth testing only index finger and great toe joints as the only likely cause of proprioceptive loss in a child is a peripheral neuropathy:
— vincristine neuropathy in leukaemics
— Guillain–Barré syndrome
— Friedreich's ataxia
— Charcot–Marie–Tooth disease and other hereditary neuropathies

Testing vibration sense in children is difficult and unlikely to give more information than the above.

The legs   Expose the legs from the groin downwards.

1. Inspection.

The same comments apply as for younger children. In particular, always look at the gait before formally examining the child's legs on the bed. The normal width of gait in children over 3 years is 10–20 cm. A very narrow gait may be a clue to the adductor spasm of a mild diplegia. A wide gait may be due to weakness or hypotonia of the legs or pelvic girdle, cerebellar dysfunction, or problems at the hip joint.

By 3 years of age a child should be able to walk on his heels, his toes, and able to stand on one leg for 5 seconds. By 4 years he can hop. From the age of 5 a child should be able to walk in a straight line for 20 steps and from the age of 7 years heel-toe walking is quite good. If there is persistent deviation or swaying, there may be abnormalities of tone, cerebellar dysfunction or a sensory neuropathy. If there are excessive associated movements of the arms, or clenching of the fists, particularly in a child over 8, the development of balance is slow.

Gaits which are uncommon in toddlers but occur in the older age group are:

— foot-drop: peroneal muscular atrophy
— dystonic gait: the effort of walking may exacerbate the slow, writhing movements of athetoid cerebral palsy, Wilson's disease and torsion dystonia.

Foot deformities and their recognized associations are discussed in the chapter on examination of the joints (Ch. 11).

2. Tone.

As for the younger child. Remember to distract the child by talking to him. Cerebral palsy is still the commonest cause of spasticity in the legs in this age group but brain tumours and cord problems are more common than in infants.

3. Power.

Again you need a very simple set of commands to test the necessary minimum of muscle groups. You must oppose the child's actions and children enjoy this 'test of strength' and will exert themselves fully.

L1, 2   As the child to lift one leg straight off the bed. 'Now keep it there while I push down against you.'

L5, S1   Now, ask the child to press the leg straight down into the bed. 'Keep it there while I pull against you.'

L3, 4   Bend the child's knee to a right angle. 'Try and straighten your leg while I push against you.'

S1   Keep the knee at a right angle. 'Now try and pull your heel towards your bottom.'

L4   Place your hand on the dorsum of the foot and extend the child's ankle. 'Pull up against my hand.'

S1, 2   Place your hand on the sole of the foot. 'Now push down against my hand.'

L5   Push on the dorsum of the big toe. 'Pull your toe towards you.'

We have given the root levels for each of the above actions. It is not worth learning the actual muscle or nerve responsible for each of these actions as isolated lesions are very rare. Remember that pyramidal weakness (upper motor neurone lesion) causes more pronounced weakness in the extensors of the arm and in the flexors of the leg, and the weakness affects movements rather than individual muscles.

(i) Cortical lesions cause contralateral paralysis, a discrete lesion in the motor cortex giving rise to a circumscribed weakness (e.g. parasagittal lesions cause a spastic diplegia).

(ii) A lesion in the internal capsule usually causes a complete contralateral hemiparesis as the descending fibres are grouped close together.

(iii) Brainstem lesions often affect both sides.

(iv) A lesion in the spinal cord gives an ipsilateral spastic paralysis below the lesion, possibly with lower motor neurone signs at the level of the lesion.

4. Reflexes.

These are elicited as for the younger child, possibly with the help of reinforcement. Always watch that the head is central when testing reflexes as the briskness of reflexes may be increased on the side to which the face is turned by the asymmetric tonic neck reflex. Children tend to have brisker reflexes in the legs than the arms. Absence of the ankle jerks only may be the first evidence of a peripheral neuropathy while preservation of the ankle jerks and absence of other deep tendon reflexes is more common in myopathies.

(i) The Babinski response.

This test may be very uncomfortable for a child. The correct method is to start near the heel, and to stroke (not gouge) your finger or an orange stick (not a key) along the lateral aspect of the sole and then medially across the ball of the foot. Splaying of the toes and dorsiflexion of the big toe is a positive response. This implies there is an upper motor neurone lesion but tells you nothing about the level of this lesion. Usually, however, the response is one of withdrawal of the foot from this unpleasant stimulus, in which case the test is uninformative (not equivocal) and there is no point in repeating it several times to the anguish of the child and of the examiners.

Testing of abdominal reflexes (T7–T12) and cremaster reflex (L1, 2) is not a routine part of the examination. If you are trying to establish the level of a cord lesion, look for a sensory level for light touch.

(ii) Clonus.

Sustained clonus is evidence of an upper motor neurone lesion although one or two beats, in the absence of any other signs may be ignored. Ankle clonus may be obtained by rapidly dorsiflexing the ankle and patellar clonus by pushing the patella downwards with the knee straight.

5. Co-ordination.

If gait, tone and power are normal, tests of co-ordination in the legs are so gross as to be a waste of time. Likewise, if gait, tone or power are abnormal, tests of co-ordination will not tell you anything new, so forget them.

6. Sensation (Fig. 8.2).

As for the arms, test only light touch and joint position sense.

Inguinal ligament   L1

Middle of anterior thigh	L2
Medial aspect of the knee	L3
Medial aspect of the calf	L4
Lateral aspect of the calf	L5
Sole of foot	S1

Only test perineal sensation if there is other evidence of a sacral cord or cauda equina lesion. The perianal skin is supplied by S3, 4, 5 and the anal sphincter may appear lax ('S2, 3, 4 keeps the faeces off the floor') or there may be obvious incontinence.

Limb girdles and trunk   The ability to test these muscle groups in children is important as the muscular dystrophies present with proximal muscle weakness. Often the initial complaint is of problems with walking, running or climbing stairs. Apart from formal testing of shoulder movements and straight leg raising as outlined above, the following may be helpful.

(i) The shoulder girdle: ask the child to mime how he would comb his hair. He may be able to do this initially but tire quickly.

(ii) The trunk: can he sit up from a supine position without the aid of his arms?

(iii) The pelvic girdle: standing from a crouching position requires powerful proximal muscles.

(iv) Gower's sign: this describes a manoeuvre used to get up off the floor, first described in boys with Duchenne's muscular dystrophy. The child will roll onto his front and then push against his thighs to straighten up, effectively climbing up his legs.

Cerebellar function   The posterior fossa is the commonest site of childhood brain tumours and an ataxic form of cerebral palsy occurs. Nystagmus, dysarthria, dysdiadochokinesia, dysmetria, intention tremor and ataxic gait have already been described. Romberg's sign is often thought to denote a cerebellar disorder but is also a sign of proprioceptive sensory loss, rare in childhood.

Romberg's sign: the child stands facing you with his feet together. Observe him for a few seconds and then ask him to close his eyes. The sign is positive if he is significantly more unsteady without visual cues.

Higher function   Tests of memory and concentration are difficult in children because of the wide variation between individuals and with age. It is more sensible to be guided by the parents and by changes in school performance (provided vision and hearing are known to be normal). However, if a child has a hemiparesis, you should know how to test parietal function.

(i) Expressive dysphasia: this is easily tested by asking the child to name simple objects such as a pen, watch etc. You can check that his vocabulary is adequate and that it is a purely expressive problem by demonstrating to the examiners that he can point to the pen and watch although he cannot name them.

(ii) Sensory perception: there may be right/left discrimination problems or gross sensory inattention for the contralateral visual field or side of the body. More subtle disturbance may be shown by testing graphaesthesia; ask the child to close his eyes and say what number you are drawing on the palm of his hand. Draw slowly, making clear strokes.

If the child has had a hemiplegia since birth due to cerebral palsy, these tests may be normal as the brain has had time to adapt. However, if the problem is recent or if the onset was after the preschool years, parietal function may be abnormal.

Always remember to measure and plot head circumference, and the parents' head circumference if the child's head is abnormally large or small.

Common neurological long cases

Cerebral palsy

Candidates who score badly on this case do so either because they fail to take an appropriate history or because they have little practical experience of the outpatient approach to long term management. The physical signs are usually obvious and rarely missed although they may be demonstrated poorly.

History

Cerebral palsy is a motor disorder as a result of non-progressive brain damage in early life. The history must address possible causes (although a definite aetiology is the exception), the impact of this disorder on the child and his family, and the steps taken to minimize the effects of the disorder.

1. Obstetric and perinatal history: the aetiology of cerebral palsy may be prenatal, perinatal or postnatal, therefore enquire about:
— infection and infectious contacts during pregnancy
— concern from ultrasound scans about the baby's growth
— vaginal bleeding during pregnancy
— high blood pressure and ankle swelling
— diabetes
— a detailed history of the labour and mode of delivery; how many weeks pregnant?
— if forceps or caesarean section were necessary, does the mother know why?
— was a paediatrician present at the delivery?
— birth weight
If the infant was admitted to the special care baby unit, then

clearly a detailed account of the infant's problems, treatment and length of stay is required. In particular, ask about:
— whether a breathing machine was necessary?
— fits
— brain scans
— exchange transfusion for jaundice

Remember, in the vast majority of cases of CP, a term infant was born by a normal delivery following a perfectly healthy pregnancy. Ask about fits, meningitis and head injuries.

2. Presentation: the commonest are
— motor delay noted by the parents
— a floppy baby, or alternatively increased tone. Hypotonia often precedes the development of spasticity
— feeding problems
— irritability
— fits
— motor delay or asymmetry detected incidentally at routine screening, or at follow-up of some other problem such as deafness or visual loss

Most children with cerebral palsy are not diagnosed definitely until after the first year of life but often some of the above features are apparent in retrospect. Many candidates mistakenly think that most cases of CP derive from the population of premature infants. In fact, less than 25% of cases have been born prematurely and although most centres closely follow all 'at risk' premature infants, most are entirely normal. A particular subgroup of CP, spastic diplegia, does however have an association with low birth weight.

3. Developmental history: only the motor milestones may have been delayed but often there are other associated problems (see below).

4. Family history. Are there any relatives with physical or mental handicap or neurological disease with the onset in early childhood?

5. Associated non-motor problems. These are common and may represent more of a handicap to the child than the motor disorder itself:
— 30% have severe learning difficulties (IQ < 50)
— 30% have moderate learning difficulties (IQ 50–70)

It is a mistake to assume that the degree of physical and mental handicap go hand-in-hand.
— 30% are epileptic
— 25% have decreased visual acuity
— 25% have a squint
— 20% have impaired hearing, usually sensorineural; hence language is often also delayed.

Therefore, ask about:
— sight, squints and spectacles
— hearing and hearing aids
— speech

— mobility
— deformity
— continence and constipation
— feeding problems
— fits and anticonvulsant medication
— behaviour problems

Finally, despite all these problems, try not to lose sight of what he actually can do rather than cannot do, the simple activities of daily living; can he dress himself, toilet himself, feed himself? There are probably particular games or sports which he prefers, in which his physical disability is less of a handicap, particularly swimming. This functional assessment is not the same as a developmental or neurological assessment.

Management   Do you know what a multidisciplinary approach is, or is it just a piece of jargon? Ask in detail about the input of the following professionals; how often does the child see them, what exactly do they do, and do the parents feel that the child derives any benefit?
— health visitor
— community nurse
— physiotherapist
— occupational therapist
— speech therapist and hearing centre
— optician and ophthalmologist
— orthopaedic surgeon
— general practitioner
— paediatrician
— teacher

Attending to the educational needs of the child is a crucial part of long term management. If the child attends a special school, some of the therapists already mentioned may be on the staff or attend regularly. However, since the Warnock report, children are encouraged to attend normal schools, especially if their handicap is purely physical. A nursery nurse may be assigned to the class to provide extra support for the child. If the child does have learning difficulties, an educational psychologist will also be involved.

Does the child have any special aids to help compensate for his handicap?
— glasses
— hearing aid
— splints
— special shoes
— wheelchair

Have any special modifications been made to the house, in particular to the toilet and bathroom or to accommodate a wheelchair? An extension may have been necessary or even a move to a new house.

What other sources of help do the parents have, financial or otherwise? Ask about:

— local self-help groups, charities and relatives
— arrangements for 'respite care' to allow the parents time for a holiday and more time with the child's siblings
— are they entitled to claim an attendance allowance (possible for children over 2 years of age) or a mobility allowance (for children over 5 years of age)?

Ask about the effect of the child's handicap on other members of the family, especially siblings.

Ask about regular medications (anticonvulsants, antispasmodics, night sedation).

Examination   The aims are to define:

1. The type of CP:

— monoplegia
— hemiplegia, usually arm > leg
— quadriplegia ('double hemiplegia'), arms > legs
— diplegia, legs > arms
— ataxic
— dyskinetic (dystonic, choreoid, athetoid)
— mixed

2. The severity: this is defined in terms of how the disability affects the child's ability to function, emphasizing what the child can do rather than cannot do.

3. Associated disabilities: a full neurological examination should be performed but particular attention should be paid to:

(i) Posture:

— Arm flexed, fisting, and leg extended in hemiplegia.
— Scissoring of spastic diplegia. When standing, his body is tilted forward and hips and knees flexed. When sitting, the back is arched.
— Windswept (gravitational) posture of very inactive child.

(ii) Tone: in 70% of CP cases, the tone is increased. This clasp-knife spasticity is classically demonstrated by extending the elbow and stretching biceps but may be much more obvious on supination of the wrist. The child may have been hypotonic initially.

(iii) Power: there may be abnormalities of tone and reflexes without obvious loss of power. However, there may then be a reduction of voluntary movements and obvious premature hand preference or exertion may precipitate an excess of involuntary, associated movements.

If power is severely reduced, contractures (or scars where they have been released) may be apparent and there may be trophic changes of dwarfing of the limb with cool, cyanosed or puffy skin.

(iv) Reflexes: brisk tendon jerks, clonus and extensor plantars may all occur in the spastic group.

(v) Gait.

Hemiplegia: look for
— the child walking on the toes of the affected side
— extension of the knee and circumduction of the leg
— shortening of the Achilles tendon and occasionally clawing of the toes

Cerebral diplegia:
— the child walks with hips and knees flexed, taking the weight on the toes. Steps are short and rotation of the body may be used to advance the leading foot.

Ataxic CP:
— a broad-based gait with arms raised to improve balance.

(vi) Cerebellar function: 10% of CP is of the ataxic type. Look for
— hypotonia
— paucity of spontaneous movements
— resting tremor of head and intention tremor of hand; ask him to hold a cup, for example
— nystagmus is very rare unless there is an associated visual problem

(vii) Involuntary movements.

Athetosis is the commonest form of dyskinesia in CP, but chorea, tremor and truncal dystonia also occur. Pharyngeal inco-ordination often leads to drooling and dysarthria. There may be associated extensor spasms and yet hypotonia, but not weakness, is very common in this group. Contractures are rare.

Common neurological short cases

The floppy infant   All young babies are floppy to a certain degree so a quantitative assessment of whether the hypotonia is pathological is required. In the majority of cases, the hypotonia is cerebral in origin. Neuromuscular disease is suggested by hypotonia accompanied by weakness, suggested by:
— paucity of movements
— a weak cry
— a poor suck
— hypoventilation and possibly paradoxical respiration (diaphragmatic weakness) or chest deformity, classically bell-shaped
— muscle wasting and winging of the scapula

Causes   1. Central.
— Down's syndrome
— Cerebral palsy (In addition to these two common causes of hypotonia, many other conditions in which mental retardation occurs are associated with hypotonia).
— Hypothyroidism

— Prader–Willi syndrome
— Some storage disorders (e.g. Niemann–Pick disease, infantile Tay–Sachs disease)

2. Nerve or muscle weakness.
Classify anatomically:

Anterior horn cell	—	spinal muscular atrophy
	—	myelomeningocoele
	—	traumatic or asphyxial cord lesions
	—	poliomyelitis
Peripheral nerve	—	Guillain–Barré syndrome
	—	lead poisoning
Neuromuscular junction	—	myasthenia gravis
Muscle	—	simple failure to thrive
	—	the muscular dystrophies
	—	dystrophia myotonica
	—	acid maltase deficiency (Pompe's disease)
	—	congenital myopathies (nemaline rod, central core etc.)

Genuine hypotonia should not be confused with increased joint laxity but both may be encountered simultaneously in conditions such as:
— osteogenesis imperfecta
— Ehlers–Danlos syndrome
— Marfan's syndrome

Examination

1. Look at the posture:
— characteristic 'frog's legs'
2. Look at the face:
— does the child have a syndrome? Shake hands with the parent (inability to relax grip in dystrophia myotonica)
— tongue fasciculation suggests spinal muscular atrophy
— protruding tongue suggests Down's syndrome, hypothyroidism or Pompe's disease
— a child who is alert and interested is unlikely to have one of the conditions associated with mental retardation
— the presence of a nasogastric tube may be due to difficulties with sucking or swallowing (e.g. cerebral disorder as in juvenile Batten's disease or bulbar palsy as in Werdnig–Hoffmann disease).
3. Lift the child:
— slips through your fingers
— rag doll on ventral suspension
— head lag on traction
4. Formally assess tone, power and reflexes as described in the previous sections of this chapter.
5. Remember to look at the genitalia (small penis in Prader–Willi syndrome) and the spine (myelomeningocoele).

Small head
Head size is closely correlated with brain size but much more loosely with intelligence. Causes of microcephaly (defined as OFC < 3rd centile):
Measure the child's head circumference and enquire about his height and weight. Plot all three on an appropriate centile chart. Measure the head circumference of all siblings and parents present.

1. Normal variation: the proportionately small child will obviously have a small head. If all measurements are more than 3 standard deviations away from the mean, consider causes of dwarfing (e.g. Russell–Silver dwarf).

2. Familial: parents with small heads often have children with small heads despite normal length and weight.

3. Pathological.

(i) Genetic (also called primary microcephaly).

Characteristic facies with sloping forehead and little brow; associated with mental retardation and may be autosomal recessive inheritance. The brain is morphologically normal on CT scan.

(ii) Secondary microcephaly due to:

(a) Perinatal insult: the face looks normal.

— congenital infection; look for hepatosplenomegaly, purpura, choroidoretinitis, deafness, heart murmur

— perinatal brain injury; normal OFC at birth but head size then falls away from the centiles. Hemiatrophy of the face or limbs may follow if the cerebral atrophy is unilateral.

(b) Fetal alcohol syndrome.

(c) Syndromes with mental retardation:

— Cornelia de Lange syndrome

— Rubenstein–Tabi syndrome

— Smith–Lemli–Opitz syndrome

(d) Syndromes with premature fusion of cranial sutures:

— Apert's syndrome

— Crouzon's syndrome

(e) Infant of mother with phenylketonuria.

Large head
Measure the head circumference and plot it on an appropriate centile chart. Measure the head circumferences of any parents or siblings present. The aetiologies of macrocephaly are usually divided into normotensive and hypertensive (look for signs of raised intracranial pressure such as bulging fontanelle, distended scalp veins, sun-setting of eyes) since this distinction determines the urgency of investigation and treatment.

1. Normotensive.

(i) Large brain (megalencephaly)

(a) Anatomical megalencephaly: excessive growth.

— Normal variants: a proportionately large baby with a large head, or a familial trait; the parents also have large heads.

— Associated with dwarfism (e.g. achondroplasia)

or gigantism (e.g. Soto's syndrome), and often developmental delay.

   (b) Metabolic megalencephaly: storage diseases, e.g.
- maple syrup urine disease.
- mucopolysaccharidoses.
- metachromatic leukodystrophy.

  (ii) Destructive malformations: absent brain replaced by fluid and often accompanied by excessive head growth
- hydranencephaly
- porencephaly
- holoprosencephaly

 (iii) Thickened calvarium of skull:

   (a) Expansion of bone marrow due to an acquired or hereditary anaemia (classically thalassaemia).

   (b) Expansion of the bone itself:
- rickets
- osteogenesis imperfecta
- osteopetrosis
- cleidocranial dysostosis

2. Hypertensive.

   (i) Chronic hydrocephalus.

   (a) Communicating:
- previous periventricular haemorrhage
- previous meningitis

   (b) Non-communicating:
- spina bifida with associated Arnold Chiari malformation
- congenital aqueduct stenosis
- Dandy Walker syndrome
- posterior fossa neoplasm

  (ii) Chronic cerebral oedema:
- benign intracranial hypertension
- vitamin A intoxication

 (iii) Chronic subdural effusion:
- following birth trauma
- following meningitis
- following child abuse

The child in a wheelchair

The commonest causes are:
- spina bifida (usually the lesion is above L2. The combination of talipes equinovarus, flexion contractures at the hip, urinary incontinence and a patulous anus is virtually pathognomoic)
- Duchenne's muscular dystrophy (by teenage)
- cerebral palsy (25% are unable to walk)

Initially, make an overall inspection:
- overall posture. The use of foam or plastic wedges suggests that the child has difficulty in maintaining his own posture, often because of hypotonia
- head size (hydrocephalus suggests spina bifida; palpate for a shunt)

— face (any dysmorphic features?)
— shake hands with the child, if old enough, and ask him to propel himself in his wheelchair to assess power and function in the arms
— indwelling urinary catheter and bag (again suggests spina bifida, or less commonly cord tumour or traumatic cord damage)
— the presence of splints, supports, gaiters, calipers and specially adapted shoes may all hint at the sites of weakness or spasticity and should be commented on

Do not attempt to examine the child in his wheelchair. Endeavour with the aid of his parents to help him onto the bed, a task which provides much information about tone and mobility. If the examiners feel that this is unnecessary, they will tell you. Ensure that his legs are completely exposed whilst keeping the genitalia covered.

In the case of a child requiring a wheelchair, the crucial distinction to be made is whether the abnormality causing the paraparesis is:
— in the head
— in the cord
— peripheral nerve or muscle disease

Examination of the legs

Candidates may be asked to 'examine the legs' of an ambulant child and the abnormal physical signs in this short case may not be neurological at all. A system for a complete examination of the lower limbs is:
— expose the legs and feet
— observe the gait
— inspect the limbs for asymmetry, scarring, deformity, and skin stigmata of neurological disease. Also look for trophic changes from denervation (shiny, cool skin with loss of hair, abnormal nail growth, possibly evidence of insensitivity to trauma) and muscle wasting or contractures
— feel for the femoral and foot pulses
— ask if either limb hurts and, if not, progress to examine quickly each of the hip, knee and ankle joints for swelling or abnormal range of movement
— if you have found no abnormalities so far, proceed to a formal neurological examination of the legs as described in the text, motor first and then sensory
— finally, do not forget to examine the spine and abdomen of a child with a paraparesis, and offer to assess anal tone although this will not be required in the exam

Mixed upper and lower motor neurone signs

The genuine combination of mixed upper and lower motor neurone signs is rare but candidates seem to find such signs with remarkable frequency and must be able to offer a few possible explanations:
1. Cord damage at the C5–T1 level, irrespective of the cause (e.g. severe scoliosis, tumour, syringomyelia) may cause lower

motor neurone signs in the arms and upper motor neurone signs in the legs.

2. The following are childhood causes of mixed upper and lower motor neurone signs in the lower limbs:

— cord compression at L3/L4 (absent knee jerks and extensor plantar reflexes). Do not confuse cord compression with cauda equina compression (causes lower motor neurone signs in the legs with 'saddle' sensory loss around the perineum and urinary incontinence)

— 'mixed' type of cerebral palsy (various combinations of hypotonia and increased reflexes)

— Friedreich's ataxia (spasticity, extensor plantars, pes cavus and absent ankle reflexes)

— metachromatic leukodystrophy (spasticity and absent tendon reflexes)

— vitamin B12 deficiency (spasticity, extensor plantars and absent ankle reflexes)

All except mixed cerebral palsy are rare so consider carefully whether you have elicited the signs correctly.

9. The developmental examination

Examiners in both the membership examination and in the DCH are encouraged to examine all candidates on their developmental assessment of children. Developmental examination assesses the acquisition of learned skills. This follows an orderly progress in a cephalic to caudal direction (there is little point in being able to walk if you cannot hold your head up and look around) and also requires the loss of the early primitive reflexes (you cannot develop finger–thumb apposition while you still have an active grasp reflex).

This can be the hardest part of the clinical to do well in and is the most difficult to prepare for. During the developmental assessment you have to be prepared to be opportunistic with the child as it is usually impossible to conduct your examination in an orderly sequence. We recommend that you talk to the examiner as you conduct your developmental assessment, in contrast to your examination of other systems (e.g. the CVS) when you assimilate important negative and positive physical signs to reach your diagnosis.

Developmental assessment is most conveniently divided into four fields; there is a sequence of development within each field, but the development in one field does not necessarily run parallel with that in another. This lack of parallelism, which has been termed dissociation, is an important concept to understand. The aim of your assessment should be to establish if development is either normal or delayed and if delayed, whether there is global delay or dissociation between fields. An example of dissociation would be a child who has impaired hearing with delayed speech in whom gross motor and fine motor development is normal.

The four fields of development are as follows:

1. Gross motor: The development of locomotion.
2. Vision and fine manipulation: The development of eye–hand control.
3. Hearing and speech: The development of language.
4. Personal and social: The integration of acquired abilities to reflect a general understanding of the environment.

Development follows an orderly sequence with each field although the rate of acquisition of abilities is very variable. The significance of delayed development within each field is also variable, with some fields of development being more important than others. Gross motor development is not as important as manipulative development, while the child's alertness, interest in surroundings and concentration are the most important factors in the assessment of mental ability. The ages at which normal children sit and walk can be very variable with some normal children not walking until 2 years of age. On the other hand, some mentally retarded children may learn to sit and walk at the usual age.

Developmental assessment requires a knowledge of the essential milestones, and failure to acquire them may be considered suspicious.

Essential milestones:

Birth	Prone: pelvis high, knees under abdomen
6 weeks	Smiles in response to maternal overtures
	prone: pelvis flat, hips extended
	Ventral suspension: head held up level with rest of body briefly
3 months	Holds rattle placed in hand
	Turns head to sound on a level with the ear
5 months	Able to go for an object and get it
6 months	Transfers an object from one hand to the other
	Chews
	Sits with hands forward for support
	Lifts head spontaneously from supine
10 months	Index finger approach to objects
	Finger–thumb apposition
	Waves 'byebye'
13 months	Casting objects
	Walks without support
	Single words
15 months	Feeds self from cup
	Domestic mimicry
	Mouthing stops
18 months	Casting stops
	Toilet control: tells mother he wants potty
2 years	Spontaneously joins two or three words together to make a sentence
	Mainly dry by day
	Cubes: tower of 6 or 7
3 years	Mainly dry by night
	Dresses and undresses fully
	Cubes: tower of 9

Primitive reflexes   These are lost as development progresses; persistence beyond these age limits reflects failure of the CNS to mature.

2 months	Palmar grip lost
	Stepping reflex lost
6 months	Moro reflex lost
	Asymmetric tonic neck reflex lost

12 months   Palmar grasp reflex lost

Babinski response becomes flexor (down-going)

5 years   Galant response (scratch along a paravertebral line, the spine curves in with concavity on the stimulated side) lost

Causes of delayed development

Delayed motor development:
    Familial feature
    Environmental factors — emotional deprivation, lack of opportunity to practise
    Mental subnormality
    Hypotonia (e.g. Down's syndrome)
    Hypertonia (e.g. cerebral palsy)
    Neuromuscular disorder (e.g. Duchenne muscular dystrophy)
    Bottom shuffling
    Blindness

Delayed speech:
    Hearing impairment
    Environmental factors — emotional deprivation
    Mental subnormality or low intelligence
    Familial feature
    Autism
    Twinning
    Cerebral palsy
    Dysphasia

Delayed sphincter control:
    Familial feature
    Mental subnormality
    Environmental factors — mismanagement of toilet training
    Physical disease   — meningomyelocoele
                       — ureterocoele
                       — ectopic ureter (female)
                       — urethral valves (male)
    Unexplained delay

Hearing

There are a number of factors which increase the chances that a child may have impaired hearing.

General:
    The parents may suspect that their child is deaf
    Behaviour problems or educational failure

Hereditary:
    Family history of deafness

Congenital:
    Down's syndrome
    Cleft palate and other congenital abnormalities of the head and neck

Non-bacterial intra-uterine infection, e.g. congenital rubella
Cystic fibrosis
Many dysmorphic syndromes, e.g.   — Hunter's
                                  — Hurler's
                                  — Kartagener
                                  — Oto–palato–digital
                                  — Treacher Collins
                                  — Waardenburg

Perinatal:
  Prematurity
  Birth asphyxia
  Ototoxic drugs taken during pregnancy or in the neonatal period
  Hyperbilirubinaemia in the neonatal period
  Cerebral palsy (particularly athetoid)

Acquired:
  Chronic otitis media or glue ear
  Delayed or defective speech
  Meningitis
  Mumps

The testing of hearing   Accurate assessment of a child's hearing can be difficult as it requires time, expertise and a quiet environment. It is, however, important to pick up deafness early as expert intervention can be very beneficial. The clinical examination is not a satisfactory setting in which to assess hearing reliably and you are unlikely to be asked to do more than go through the motions.

The method of assessment is determined by the age of the child.

Screening for deafness   Screening at 8 months:
The distraction test is used by health visitors (see below).

Screening at 3 years:
Assessment of language development (the child should be speaking in short sentences) and the Stycar picture hearing test.

Screening at 7 years.
Pure-tone audiometry using a set level (usually 20 dB) at a number of frequencies.

Measurement of hearing   Neonate:
The infant should startle or quieten to a loud stimulus (e.g. a clap). Formal measurement requires auditory evoked responses.

6–18 months: The distraction test
The infant sits on the parent's knee facing the observer who raises the child's level of interest. The source of interest is

removed and the tester introduces a calibrated sound of known intensity and frequency 30–45 cm from the ear at an angle of 45° on a level with the ear. Suitable sounds are PSS for high tones and OOO for low tones, or a Manchester rattle. Avoid blowing into the ear. By 6 months the child turns the head to the side at which the sound is heard. It is the person who is visually distracting the child who must say if the child responded.

2 years:

By 2 years children can be conditioned to respond to a sound with play material (e.g. a brick into a bucket or a development board). The stimulus can be a measured 'go' or 'sss' or a pure tone, and both sides can be tested. If using a vocal stimulus the mouth should be covered. Speech audiometry using specific phonetically matched toys can be used from about 2 years in the co-operative child.

3 years:

By 3 years most children will be able to co-operate with pure-tone audiometry. Headphones are used to deliver a signal at a known frequency and intensity and the child signals when they hear the signal by, for example, dropping a cube in a bucket. This requires considerable expertise to maintain the child's interest and concentration. Impedance audiometry is an objective physical measurement of the compliance of the tympanic membrane. This method detects the presence of fluid in the middle ear causing conductive hearing loss and can be used in infants from about 6 months.

Vision   There are a number of factors which should alert you to the possibility that a child has a visual defect.

General:
   The presence of nystagmus (roving)
   Behaviour problems or educational failure
   Family history of blindness, squint or amblyopia

Congenital:
   Congenital rubella
   Craniostenosis

Perinatal:
   Prematurity
   Severe pre-eclampsia: risk of myopia
   Hydrocephalus
   Cerebral palsy
   Ophthalmia neonatorum

Before testing vision inspect the eye for:
   Lens opacity
   Presence of red reflex

Ptosis (may be bilateral)
Strabismus (see later section)
Normal pupillary responses

Testing visual acuity   4 weeks:
The infant should fix on his mother's face.

6 weeks:
Follows an object 90 cm away through an angle of 90°. A 4 cm red ball or pen torch are suitable objects.

3 months: ·
Follows an object 90 cm away for 180° while lying supine.

10 months:
Can go for an object the size of a raisin lying in the palm of your hand and pick it up between finger and thumb. Test with each eye covered. By one year they can pick up individual 'hundreds and thousands'.

2–3 years:
Test with miniature toys. Use the following toys: chair, doll, car, plane, spoon, knife and fork. The majority of children over 2 years of age can identify all seven toys. The procedure involves familiarizing the child with all the toys and then, at a distance of 3 m from the child, asking the child 'What's this?'. If the child cannot speak intelligibly then he should be given a duplicate set of toys of a different colour from those being shown and encouraged to indicate which toy is the same as the examiner's. Test both eyes and then each in turn.

3 years:
After the age of 3 years you can use the Stycar matching letters. The first letters to be learnt by a child are V, O, X, H and T, and later A, U, I and C. Once he is familiar with the procedure, the child matches letters in his own set with letters held up by the examiner at a distance of 3 m. The size of the letters decreases and visual acuity can be assessed. Test both eyes and then each in turn. Near vision is tested in the same way using a near vision chart at about 46 cm. Normal vision between 3 and 5 years approximates R: 6/8, L: 6/8.

From 5 years:
By 5 years most children are able to read the Snellen charts sitting in front of a mirror at 3 m. The Ishihara plates can also be used in boys from this age to test for colour vision.

Squint   Definition:
A squint (strabismus) is present if one of the eyes is not directed towards the object under scrutiny. A squint may be paralytic or concomitant (non-paralytic).

Aetiology:
1. Paralytic: cranial nerve palsies of the 3 (divergent), 4 or

6 (convergent) cranial nerves. A 6th nerve palsy may be associated with raised intracranial pressure. Paralytic squints are common in children with cerebral palsy and mental retardation.

2. Concomitant: A non-paralytic squint may be due to a refractive error, eye disease or failure to develop binocular vision. Eye conditions which may present with a squint include a corneal scar, cataract, retinopathy of prematurity and retinoblastoma.

Assessment of the child with a squint:

1. Check visual acuity of each eye independently.

2. Observe the position of the child's eyes. If a paralytic squint is present the angle subtended by the eyes will vary with the direction of gaze.

3. Look at the corneal reflections of a bright light held in front of the eyes. The position of the reflections on the eyes should be symmetrical.

4. Cover tests: there are two types which may be used to reveal a squint.

— Cover/uncover test: One eye is covered and the other eye is observed. If the uncovered eye moves to fix on the object there is a squint which is present all the time — a manifest squint. The test should be carried out by covering each eye in turn.

— Alternate cover test: If the cover/uncover test is normal, which indicates that no manifest squint is present, the alternate cover test should be used. The occluder is moved to and fro between the eyes and if the eye which has been uncovered moves then a latent squint is present.

5. Careful examination of the optic fundus.

The purpose of screening for squints is to detect refractive problems, diagnose underlying eye disease and prevent amblyopia (the suppression of vision in a structurally and functionally normal eye).

Serious visual impairment in children

Each year in the UK more than 450 children under 15 years of age are registered blind or partially sighted. The importance of recognizing visually handicapped children is threefold:

1. Early treatment may prevent visual disability or reduce its severity.

2. Genetic counselling, medical and social support can be provided as required.

3. Some of the causes of blindness are associated with systemic disease.

The causes of visual impairment in children can be divided as follows:

Cataract
Optic nerve pathology
Retinal pathology
Trauma to any part of the eye

Albinism
Glaucoma
Nystagmus
Delayed visual maturation
Visual loss before the age of 2 years is usually accompanied by 'roving' eye movements, persistent hand regard, lack of blink to menace and nystagmus.

Cataract   Bilateral opacification of the lens accounts for up to 30% of visually handicapped babies. The diagnosis is suggested by absence of the normal pupillary red reflex.
The three main causes of congenital cataract are:
Familial
Secondary to prenatal infections
Associated with prematurity
Other conditions associated with cataract are:
Down's syndrome
Children on continuous corticosteroid treatment
Trauma to the eye
Diabetes mellitus
Myotonic dystrophy
Hypoparathyroidism
Lowe's syndrome
Wilson's disease
Galactokinase deficiency
Galactosaemia
Early removal of cataracts with optical correction can offer an excellent visual prognosis.

Optic nerve pathology   Optic nerve pathology blinds as many children as cataract but is less amenable to treatment. Most causes of optic atrophy are inherited. The optic disc of normal babies is pale and can be difficult to distinguish from optic atrophy.

Causes:
May be associated with cerebral palsy.
Septo–otic dysplasia (absence of septum pellucidum and associated with hypopituitarism).
Intracranial tumours and hydrocephalus.
Leber's hereditary optic atrophy, which rarely presents in young children.

Retinal pathology   Retinopathy of prematurity (ROP) is the predominant cause which may also be associated with cataracts. The condition is more common in premature babies weighing <1500 g.
Other causes include:
Leber's amaurosis, an autosomal recessive disorder which presents as a congenital retinitis pigmentosa.
Retinoblastoma: The most important reason for hospital evaluation of any child with a visual defect, retinoblastoma has an incidence of 1 in 18 000 live births and will present initially with a squint alone in about 33% of cases.

Toxoplasmosis, which causes the typical 'clock-face' macula scar.

Glaucoma Congenital glaucoma or bupthalmos presents with globe enlargement, clouding of the cornea and photophobia. Associated conditions include Sturge–Weber syndrome and aniridia (absence of iris bilaterally).

Nystagmus (see also Ch. 8) Visual loss before the age of 2 is usually accompanied by nystagmus; however, nystagmus due to unstable ocular fixation will lead to a reduction in measured visual acuity.

Developmental screening

Screening at 6 weeks   History:
Full birth history including complications of pregnancy
Medical history to date
Age of onset of smiling and vocalization
Response to sound
Sucking and swallowing difficulties

Examination:
Is the facial appearance normal?
Is the anterior fontanelle normotensive?
Examine the eyes for squint, red reflex and nystagmus
Examine the spine
Hold in ventral suspension
Place in the prone position
Pull to sitting position from supine
Test weight bearing
Examine the mouth for candidiasis and palate to exclude a cleft
Measure head circumference and plot on chart with weight and length
Examine hips for congenital dislocation
Test reflexes if any doubt about muscle tone or posture
Test primitive reflexes (certainly not essential)

Screening at 6 months   History: As for 6 week screen, plus age of onset of
Holding a rattle placed in the hand
Turning head to sound
Reaching out and getting object
Sitting
Chewing

Examination:
Is the facial appearance and expression normal?
Is the anterior fontanelle normotensive?
Examine the eyes for squint, red reflex and nystagmus
Notice alertness and interest in surroundings
Examine the spine

Feel the abdomen and examine the external genitalia, palpating for descent of the testes in boys

Using one inch cubes observe nature of grasp and observe for ability to transfer objects

Pull to sit from supine noting particularly head control

Note sitting ability

Test weight bearing

Assess muscle tone and reflexes if indicated

Measure head circumference and plot on chart with weight and length

Test the hearing

Examine hips for congenital dislocation

Screening at 10 months   History: As for 6 month screen, plus age of onset of

Crawling

Creeping

Standing holding on

Pulling self to sit and stand

Waves 'bye'

Helps to dress

Any words with meaning

Examination: As for 6 months but with the following additions:

Offer a raisin in the palm of your hand or his mother's hand and, covering each eye in turn, observe for index finger approach and finger–thumb apposition

Test sitting ability

Screening at 2 years   History: As before, plus age of onset of

Joining words together to make a sentence

Is he dry day and/or night?

Walking alone

Ability to dress and feed himself

How many words he says with meaning

Does he understand everything said to him and does he come when called from another room?

Examination:

Measure height, weight and head circumference and plot on chart

Observe facial expression, alertness, interest in surroundings and speech

General physical examination including hip abduction

Inspect the eyes for squint, lens opacity and nystagmus

Observe gait when walking

By 2 years he should be able to construct a tower of six or seven cubes

Test hearing

Test visual acuity

10. The skin

The dermatological cases you are most likely to see are those which are not uncommonly found on acute paediatric wards (e.g. eczema, drug rash, erythema multiforme, purpura), which may be incidental to the reason for admission; or chronic cases which can be arranged easily in advance of the examination day (e.g. psoriasis, dermatitis herpetiformis). Alternatively, if you are taking the exam in a large centre or children's hospital in which there is a specific paediatric dermatology ward or infectious diseases unit, you may see some very rare rashes indeed! Many of the conditions mentioned in this chapter are extremely rare in general paediatric practice but you will be expected to suggest a list of differentials for a number of common dermatological presentations, such as generalized maculo-papular rash, an itchy rash and a circumscribed patch of decreased pigmentation.

Examination of the skin as a system includes inspection of the mucous membranes, hair, nails and teeth. Indeed, examination of the skin is dependent on powers of observation with the aid of palpation of the lesions, so always ensure that a prepubertal child is completely undressed. Congenital variants are discussed in Chapter 12 on the neonate and the skin abnormalities associated with the neurophakomatoses are discussed in Chapter 8 on the nervous system and Chapter 13 on common exam syndromes.

Absence of hair: Localized:
— alopecia areata (look for exclamation mark hairs at the edge of the patch). The cause is unknown.
— trichillomania (hair pulling)
— ringworm
— short occipital hair may occur in a child with motor delay who is left supine for much of the time
Generalized:
— alopecia totalis may develop from areata
— cytotoxic therapy
— recent neurosurgery or cranial irradiation
— ectodermal dysplasia; look for associated dental hypoplasia and absent nails in this rare sex-linked recessive disorder.

Abnormalities of the hair: — coarse facial hair from chronic phenytoin therapy
— white forelock of Waardenburg's syndrome

— bushy eyebrows of Cornelia de Lange syndrome
— kinky hair of Menkes' syndrome

Abnormalities of the nails:
— pitted nails in psoriasis
— Beau's lines (a transverse ridge corresponding to arrested nail growth during a severe illness)
— paronychia is common in newborn infants
— fungal infection may cause separation of the nail from the bed (onycholysis)
— splinter haemorrhages under the nail are seen in bacterial endocarditis
— deformed nails in epidermolysis bullosa
— absent nails in ectodermal dysplasia
— koilonychia (spoon-shaped nails) is a sign of chronic severe iron deficiency anaemia and is rarely seen nowadays
— leuchonychia (diffusely white nails) is a result of chronic hypoalbuminaemia in nephrotic syndrome and liver disease.
— white spots on the nails are a normal variant.

Describing a skin lesion

Dermatologists make their subject more difficult than it need be by couching their terminology in Latin phrases and using confusing classifications. For the paediatrician, the best approach is to describe exactly what you see in plain English.

The skin is the only organ visible to the outside world and is the interface with both our physical and social environment. Try to empathize with the child, anticipating how the stigma of an abnormality of the skin may affect him.

Define a skin abnormality as follows:

1. The site and whether single or multiple, and where most dense (centrifugal or centripetal).

2. The size and whether uniform or varied. 'Morbilliform' and 'rubelliform' are used to describe rashes with macules similar to those in measles or rubella respectively.

3. The colour, which again may vary. The colour of an abnormality may be strikingly different from the surrounding skin, e.g. a haemangioma. Alternatively, there may be more subtle variations in the shade of flesh colour:
— vitiligo (depigmented patches)
— lentigines (brown spots, as in the acronymous leopard syndrome)

Hypopigmentation and hyperpigmentation are discussed in more detail below (for café au lait spots and axillary freckling, see Chs. 8 and 13).

4. The shape. Common usages are:
— discoid
— nummular (coin-shaped)
— confluent
— multiforme (simply means 'of many shapes' and is not confined to the target lesions of erythema multiforme)

— target lesions
— annulare
— umbilicated (having a central depression, as in the lesions of molluscum contagiosum, but not on a stalk as many candidates think)
    5. The feel. Common terms are:
— macule (flush with the skin)
— papule (raised above the surrounding skin)
— marginatum (the edge is raised, as in erythema marginatum)
— lichenified (thickened)
— icthyotic (dry and scaling)
Many rashes are itchy but very few are painful or infectious. Palpation of a skin lesion is all too often forgotten.

Hypopigmentation

May be localized or generalized:

Local:
— previous inflammation (e.g. herpes zoster) burn or scar
— vitiligo (usually bilateral and symmetrical, associated with alopecia areata and autoimmune disease)
— tuberose sclerosis
— pityriasis versicolor (a fungal infection)
— pityriasis alba (usually cheeks and sometimes upper arms, accompanied by scaling)

General:
— albinism (pink pupils, blue irides and white hair)
— phenylketonuria (blonde hair and blue eyes)
— hypopituitarism (short stature and micropenis)

Hyperpigmentation

May be localized or generalized:

Local:
— previous inflammation
— pigmented naevus or melanoma
— café au lait spots in neurofibromatosis and Albright's syndrome (polyostotic fibrous dysplasia and sexual precocity in females). More than six, each more than 1.5 cm diameter, are considered significant.
— Peutz–Jegher syndrome (pigmented spots in or around the mouth often associated with gastrointestinal bleeding; autosomal dominant)
— chronic phenytoin therapy (also gum hypertrophy and coarse, hirsute facies)
— leopard syndrome (lentigines, ECG abnormalities, ocular defects, pulmonary stenosis, abnormal genitalia, retarded growth, deafness)

General:
— racial or suntan

— haemosiderosis (e.g. multiple transfusions for thalassaemia)
— Addison's disease
— primary biliary cirrhosis

Itchy rashes

May indicate:
— eczema
— psoriasis
— dermatitis herpetiformis (associated with coeliac disease)
— ringworm (a confusing misnomer since tinea capitis, tinea corporis and tinea pedis are all fungal infections)
The following are unlikely to be seen in an exam:
— urticaria and insect bites
— scabies (itches where the mite burrows)
— pityriasis rosea (herald patch)
— both tinea capitis (fungal) and pediculosis capitis (the nits, or eggs, of lice) cause itching of the scalp
Visual clues suggesting that a skin condition is itchy are the presence of excoriation, the wearing of mitts and the Koebner phenomenon.

The Koebner phenomenon

Itching or trauma to previously unaffected skin results in fresh lesions:
— psoriasis
— lichen planus
Infective skin lesions such as warts and impetigo can be spread by scratching but this is not the true Koebner phenomenon.

Palms and soles

Lesions which may affect the palms or soles are:
— erythema multiforme. This is the only palmar lesion you are likely to see in the exam as cases of Stevens–Johnson syndrome are not uncommon on general paediatric wards.
— vesicles of hand, foot and mouth disease (Coxsackie A)
— desquamation of Kawasaki's disease or following streptococcal infection. Desquamation may follow friction (common blister, e.g. on the heel from new shoes), and separation of the epidermis (Nikolsky's sign) is a feature of scalded skin syndrome in the newborn. This staphylococcal condition, also known as Lyell's or Ritter's disease, is unlikely to be seen in the exam.
— pustular psoriasis
— pompholyx, a bullous form of eczema
— malignant melanoma

Lesions which 'never' affect palms or soles are:
— benign naevus (common 'mole')
— sebaceous cyst
— lipoma

Blisters, vesicles and bullae

These are all fluid-filled lesions. By convention, a bulla is larger than a vesicle and a blister is the result of friction or a burn. A vesicle which contains pus is a pustule; a boil is a collection of pus in the skin but not preceded by a clear vesicle. The differential diagnosis depends on the age of the child:

Neonate:
— bullous impetigo is due to staphylococcal skin infection whereas the rarer scalded skin syndrome is due to a staphylococcal exotoxin
— herpes simplex
— epidermolysis bullosa. The autosomal recessive forms are severe whereas the autosomal dominant forms are milder. Look for old scars and nail deformities
— incontinentia pigmenti affects only girls. Look for old scars, hyperpigmented whorls and dental abnormalities.

Child:
— insect bites
— chickenpox
— herpes zoster
— herpes simplex
— dermatitis herpetiformis (usually confined to buttocks or genitalia)
— erythema multiforme (rarely)

Haemorrhages in the skin

These are defined by size:
— petechiae are 1 mm or less in diameter
— purpuric spots are 2–10 mm in diameter
— ecchymoses are larger bruises
— a haematoma is a haemorrhage large enough to produce a tender elevation of the skin

Haemorrhages into the skin do not blanche with pressure which helps distinguish these from telangiectases and erythema which are due to dilated skin blood vessels. Purpura due to a vasculitis (as in Henoch–Schönlein purpura and meningococcaemia) may be palpable whereas purpura due to thrombocytopenia is usually flush with the surrounding skin.

Aetiological classification of skin haemorrhage

Virchow's triad specifies that there are three components of the coagulation system (vascular endothelium, platelets and clotting factors) and that an abnormality of any of these may result in haemorrhage.

Vascular abnormalities:
— Henoch–Schönlein purpura
— meningococcal septicaemia
— increased fragility
  • chronic steroid effect
  • Ehlers–Danlos syndrome
  • vitamin C deficiency (scurvy)

Thrombocytopenia:
  Increased consumption of platelets:
— idiopathic thrombocytopenic purpura
— iso-immune thrombocytopenia (rare cause of thrombocytopenia in the newborn, analogous to iso-immune haemolysis of red cells)
— haemolytic uraemic syndrome
— disseminated intravascular coagulation
— hypersplenism
— Wiskott–Aldrich syndrome (thrombocytopenia, eczema and increased susceptibility to infection; affects boys only)
— Kasabach–Merritt syndrome (large cavernous haemangiomas in skin or abdominal viscera)
  Decreased production of platelets:
— leukaemia
— cytotoxic drugs
— aplastic anaemia due to certain drugs, familial (Fanconi's anaemia) or idiopathic
— thrombocytopenia absent radius syndrome

Defective platelet function:
— von Willebrand's disease (qualitative platelet defect and factor VIII deficiency). An autosomal dominant condition with variable expression.

Abnormal clotting:
— Haemophilia A (sex-linked recessive disorder due to factor VIII deficiency)
— Haemophilia B (sex-linked disorder due to factor IX deficiency. Also known as Christmas disease)
— von Willebrand's disease (see above)
— haemorrhagic disease of the newborn (vitamin K deficiency)
— chronic liver disease (vitamin K deficiency)
— too much warfarin (antagonises vitamin K)

Common long case

Eczema   First, a word of clarification about terminology. Eczema and dermatitis are synonymous, describing a red itchy rash which may be dry or moist and sometimes raised and thickened. However, dermatitis is used more often to describe the skin abnormality in adults in whom it is often a reaction to a specific environmental trigger. The term atopic eczema is used for the condition, commonest in early childhood and often resolving by puberty, in which the aetiology of the skin disorder remains unclear but is part of a wider constitutional atopy. Although specific allergens may give positive skin tests, exposure to these seems to bear little relevance to clinical fluctuations in the disease.

History 1. When did the rash first appear? An onset after the age of 2 years may carry a worse prognosis, and an onset before the age of 3 months is unusual for truly atopic eczema. It is more likely that the eczema was preceded by a monilial or ammoniacal nappy rash or by seborrheic dermatitis.

2. Where did the rash first appear? Infantile eczema usually affects the cheeks and limb flexures. If the initial lesions were confined to extensor surfaces, and particularly if the first attack was not until school age, consider psoriasis.

3. Was the infant breast- or bottle-fed? There is some evidence that avoidance of cow's milk protein early in life protects against later atopy and therefore the incidence is less in children who were breastfed. However, the relationship between cow's milk protein and the risk of atopy is not dose-dependent and breastfeeding must be completely exclusive until the age of 3 months to confer this advantage. Some would argue that the breastfeeding mother should also be on a diet free of cow's milk protein.

4. Must the child adhere to any dietary restrictions, and how secure is the foundation for this practice?

5. Does the child also suffer from asthma or allergic rhinitis, seasonal ('hay fever') or otherwise?

6. Is there a family history of eczema, asthma or hay fever? First degree relatives have, or have had, some form of atopy in over 50% of cases.

7. How has the eczema affected the child's self-image and has it resulted in teasing at school? Severe eczema is very trying for the parents as well as the child, so ask about sleepless nights, frequency of hospital visits and admissions, and fears about the cosmetic outlook.

Management Ask specifically about the following measures:
— an emollient, such as aqueous cream, applied frequently to prevent the skin drying
— emulsifying ointment instead of soap
— reducing the frequency of baths and adding oil to the bath water
— avoiding woollens and synthetic fibres next to the skin
— avoiding 'biological' washing powders for clothes
— measures to reduce itching:
  trimming fingernails and toenails
  cotton mitts
  bandaging of affected limbs
  calamine lotion or coal tar ointment (especially for lichenified lesions)
  night sedation
— the use of topical corticosteroids. The order of increasing potency is:
  hydrocortisone

clobetasone butyrate (eumovate)
betamethasone (betnovate)
clobetasone proprionate (dermovate)
— the use of topical or systemic antibiotics for secondary infection
— atopic eczema is not a contra-indication to any of the standard immunizations given to children in the UK; this includes the measles vaccine

Examination Patches of eczema are usually:
— red
— itchy
— raised
— excoriated
— of different sizes
— symmetrical

Eczema may be dry or weeping. There is a prediliction for the skin creases and the face but in severe cases the rash may be very widespread and accompanied by generalized lymphadenopathy. Look for local (thin skin or striae) and systemic side-effects of steroid therapy, and for evidence of bacterial superinfection (yellow scabs or pustules).

Always examine the respiratory system carefully for any signs of chronic or active asthma.

Always plot the child's height and weight on an appropriate centile chart as severe eczema can adversely affect growth, not least because of severe and inappropriate dietary restrictions.

Purpura Purpura is easily recognized and is a common physical sign in the short cases. Below is an easily remembered scheme for differentiating the aetiology.

This is not meant to be a comprehensive list of the causes of purpura but these are the commonest causes to be met in the exam.

	Normal platelets	Low platelets
'Nice'	Henoch–Schönlein purpura Whooping cough Vitamin C deficiency	Idiopathic thrombocytopenic purpura
'Nasty'	Non-accidental injury Meningococcal septicaemia (purpura is classically necrotic) Clotting disorders	Acute lymphoblastic leukaemia Haemolytic uraemic syndrome Disseminated intravascular coagulation Hypersplenism

11. The limbs and joints

Clinically, the correct sequence for assessing joint pathology is 'look, feel, move, X-ray'. Whilst the benefit of radiographs is not usually available at postgraduate exams (although they are sometimes used during short cases in the DCH), this approach is still valid.

Looking Quickly take note of the general appearance of the child:
— thriving?
— any bandages, splints, plaster of Paris or traction?
— in a wheelchair?
— other deformities (e.g. kyphoscoliosis or contractures)?
Ask whether any part of the limb is painful and what exacerbates the pain. Although technically this is part of the history, it is an essential enquiry to make before touching the limb. Pain in a joint may cause spasm of adjacent muscles, although this is not usually detectable clinically, and the joint is usually held in midflexion as this position places minimum tension on the joint capsule. Pain in the knee may be referred from the hip joint and pain in the hip/thigh from the lower back. There may be obvious erythema and swelling around an acutely inflamed joint although you are more likely to see a chronic arthropathy in the exam.

A chronically painful joint may be frankly deformed or there may be associated wasting of muscles acting about that joint (disuse atrophy). Look for trophic skin changes (see Ch. 8).

Feeling Palpate the joint for skin temperature and tenderness, starting from an area of normal skin some distance away from the affected joint for comparison. Temperature is best judged with the back of the hand. Tenderness is what the child feels as a direct response to palpation, as opposed to pain which may be present all the time. Anticipate the possibility of tenderness by starting with very gentle palpation and watching the child's expression; a heavy-handed approach looks inexperienced and unsympathetic.

Palpable swelling may be due to an effusion (more likely with an acute arthropathy) or synovial swelling (more likely with a chronic arthropathy) or both. The most common site at which an effusion is detectable is the knee joint. Use the palm of the left hand to massage the fluid down from the synovial space above the patella and, maintaining pressure with the left hand, press with the thumb of the right hand over the medial aspect of the knee. The tense, fluid-filled swelling should be palpable 'bimanually' and this technique is much more sensitive, and a lot less painful, than a positive 'patellar tap'.

Moving   Active movements (i.e. by the child) should always be attempted before passive movements (i.e. by you). It is impossible to memorize the normal range of movements at every joint, especially since it varies with age and sex, but much can be learned by comparing left and right limbs or comparing an older child to yourself:
elbow: 140°
wrist: 180°
knee: 140°
It is important to decide whether joint movement is limited by pain, contracture, or even a neurological spasticity.

Infection is, of course, the commonest cause of an acute monoarthropathy but in any child with monoarthropathy or polyarthropathy, acute or chronic, show the examiners that you are aware of possible systemic aetiologies:

Trauma !

— juvenile chronic arthritis. Offer to examine the eyes for iridocyclitis in an older child; hepatosplenomegaly and lymphadenopathy in a younger child
— haemarthrosis. Look for bruising or petechiae which suggest haemophilia. Ask about trauma
— Henoch–Schönlein purpura. Look at the legs and buttocks for palpable purpura (vasculitis)
— rheumatic fever. Feel for rheumatic nodules, listen for a cardiac murmur, and ask about any recent sore throat

Foot deformities   Pes planus:
— benign flat feet
— Marfan's syndrome
— cerebral palsy
Pes cavus: a highly arched foot may be associated with:
— spina bifida occulta
— diastometamyelia (weakness and sensory impairment in the legs, possibly bladder problems and unequal lower limb growth due to spinal tethering)
— Friedreich's ataxia (cerebellar ataxia, pyramidal tract signs, dorsal column sensory loss and scoliosis)
— Charcot–Marie–Tooth disease (peroneal muscular atrophy and absent leg reflexes)
Talipes equino varus:
— spina bifida cystica
— Peroneal muscular atrophy (Charcot–Marie–Tooth disease; 'champagne bottle' muscle wasting in the legs and dorsal column sensory loss)

Neonatal hip examination

In the United Kingdom, every newborn infant undergoes a screening examination for congenital dislocation of the hips (CDH). Despite this, children continue to present at an older age with undiagnosed CDH but what remains unclear is whether the CDH was missed during the screening exam or whether the hips became dislocated later, i.e. not every case may be strictly 'congenital'. It remains for large trials to be carried out to demonstrate whether ultrasound examination in the newborn period can reduce the incidence of these late presentations.

In the newborn the classic signs of dislocation, such as asymmetrical skin folds, limited abduction, and an apparently shortened femur (Galeazzo's sign), are usually absent; these signs are secondary and do not usually develop until the age of 6 weeks. CDH in the immediate newborn period is diagnosed by using two 'provocation manoeuvres' to demonstrate that the femoral head can be dislocated and then lifted back into the acetabulum.

Lie the infant supine on a flat hard surface and remove the nappy. Start with the infant's knees together and the hips and knees held flexed at 90° with the candidate's thumbs on the medial condyles of each femur and the tips of the middle fingers on the greater trochanters of each femur. Now attempt to push the hips posteriorly (down into the bed); if you feel a 'click', the head of the femur has dislocated and Barlow's sign is positive. Now, keeping your grip unchanged, lift the femoral heads forward with the middle fingers while you abduct the thighs with your thumbs. If you feel a definite 'clunk' (the femoral head returning to the acetabulum) the dislocation is reducible and Ortolani's sign is positive. These signs remain positive in CDH up to 6–8 weeks of age, but thereafter negative provocation tests do not exclude CDH as the hip may be permanently and irreducibly dislocated. The secondary signs discussed above then become much more significant.

CDH affects girls and the left hip more commonly. If CDH is present, ask about family history and breech delivery, and look for a neural tube defect, torticollis and talipes calcaneovalgus, which are recognized associations.

Examination of the spine

The examination of the spine of a neonate is discussed elsewhere (see Ch. 12). The features associated with spina bifida are discussed in Chapter 8 on the neurological system.

Scoliosis

Reference has been made to scoliosis in the chapters on the respiratory and neurological systems. Inspect from behind with the child standing. The convention is to describe a curvature by the direction of the convexity (e.g. convex to the right) and if one shoulder is higher than the other, it is the shoulder on the convex side which is elevated. Remain behind the child and ask him to touch his toes. A postural scoliosis will disappear whereas a fixed scoliosis will persist and there is a gibbus, a hump due to increased convexity of the underlying ribs (secondary to rotation of the vertebrae), on the side of the convexity.

Postural scoliosis (80%):
— idiopathic (usually adolescent girls)
— unilateral muscle spasm secondary to pain
— unequal leg length
Structural scoliosis (20%):
— idiopathic
— unilateral muscle weakness (rarer since the decline in polio but muscular dystrophy may result in scoliosis)
— congenital abnormality of the vertebrae e.g. hemivertebrae
— osteogenesis imperfecta
— neurofibromatosis
— Marfan's syndrome
— postirradiation

Scoliosis is associated with:
— Sprengel's shoulder. One scapula is fixed in a high position due to failure of descent during fetal development. There is limited abduction of the shoulder and there may be hypoplasia of the shoulder girdle muscles. There may also be a cervical rib (and therefore brachial plexus compression).
— Klippel–Feil syndrome. The fundamental defect is fusion of the cervical spine. This results in a short neck, low hairline and webbing of the skin of the neck (differential diagnosis is Turner's syndrome). There is restricted neck movement and sometimes torticollis. There may also be cervical spina bifida and thoracic hemivertebrae (and hence root or cord compression).

Common long case

Child with a limp   An acute limp is usually the result of pain, especially joint pain, occurring anywhere from the toe to the spine. The commonest causes are:
— malignancy, particularly acute lymphoblastic leukaemia
— local trauma
— irritable hip (usually boys)
— reactive viral arthritis
Less common are:
— juvenile rheumatoid arthritis
— bacterial arthritis
— osteomyelitis
— Osgood–Schlatter disease (usually boys)
— Chondromalacia patellae (usually girls)
— Perthe's disease (usually boys)
— slipped femoral epiphysis

Juvenile rheumatoid arthritis and Perthe's disease are probably the most common causes encountered in the MRCP exam.

A chronic limp is more likely to be seen in the postgraduate examinations than an acute limp and is more likely to be the result of a deformity or weakness rather than pain. Clubfoot is one of the commonest congenital abnormalities, usually talipes equinovarus (ankle inverted and plantar flexed).

Are the legs of equal length? (see Fig. 11.1.) There may be scoliosis due to pelvic tilt but to assess leg length properly, the child must lie on a flat surface and leg length is measured from anterior superior iliac spine to medial malleolus with a tape measure. Causes of a true difference in leg length are:

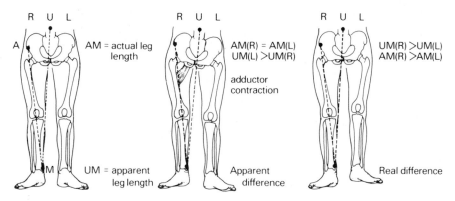

Fig. 11.1 Real and apparent differences in leg length (Reproduced with permission from Milner A D, Hull D (eds) 1984 Hospital paediatrics. Churchill Livingstone, Edinburgh.)

— previous trauma or bony surgery
— severe hemiparesis (this can also cause an apparent difference in leg length because adductor spasm causes pelvic tilt)
— osteogenesis imperfecta (look for blue sclerae and hyperextensible joints)
— Ollier's disease
— polyostotic fibrous dysplasia (café au lait patches and sexual precocity in girls)
— hemihypertrophy usually results in a difference in girth but may also alter length. Associations are:
    idiopathic
    Wilm's tumour (look for associated aniridia)
    neurofibromatosis
    arteriovenous malformation
    diastometamyelia

Having demonstrated the limp and measured leg length, examine the legs for deformities, surgical scars, rashes and joint swelling and proceed to assess range of movements at ankle, knee and hip joints after enquiring about the site of any pain.

12. The neonate

Examination
General observations

1. Is he thriving?

2. Was this infant born prematurely?

3. Is he dysmorphic? Dysmorphology is much more difficult in the neonate than in the older child and only definite abnormalities should be noted. 'Soft signs' are usually because he looks like his parents!

4. Skin:

— pallor

— plethora (think of small for gestational age (SGA) and infant of a diabetic mother)

— jaundice (yellow/orange is usually due to a haemolytic jaundice whereas khaki/green is a feature of obstructive jaundice. However, this is not reliable and you should say that you would always measure the bilirubin, conjugated and unconjugated)

— cyanosis (see Ch. 5)

— nails and umbilical stump for chronic meconium staining
Normal variants in skin markings:

(i) 'Stork bites'

— red macules

— often nape of neck or forehead

— most fade spontaneously

(ii) 'Mongolian spot'

— blue or grey macule, sometimes mutiple

— lumbosacral or buttocks

— majority of Oriental, Asian, African and Caribbean infants

— most fade spontaneously

Naevi:

(i) 'Strawberry naevus' (capillary or cavernous haemangioma)

— raised red lesion

— can occur anywhere on the body

— most regress spontaneously

(ii) 'Port wine stain'

— red to purple flat lesion

— can occur anywhere on the body

— may be unilateral (see Sturge–Weber syndrome, Chapter 8)

— does not disappear

5. Maturity: you must be familiar with the general principles of the Dubowitz examination, although you would not be expected to have memorized every detail. You are unlikely

to see the thin gelatinous skin of a newly born premature infant. Postmature infants often have wrinkled or desquamating skin, particularly over the creases of the hands; desquamation may also occur with staphylococcal infections.

Having taken a look at the infant overall, the easiest way of examining the newborn is from head to toe, rather than by system. Particular points to note in the neonate will be emphasized and material included in the chapters on individual systems will not be duplicated.

The face
— Flaring of the alar nasi is a sign of respiratory distress.
— Bruising and forceps marks. Marked facial asymmetry suggests facial nerve palsy.
— Ears for maturity, bruising, pre-auricular tags and position (see Ch. 13 for definition of low-set ears).

The eyes
— Look for hypertelorism and the angle of the palpebral fissures (see Ch. 13). Do not comment unless definitely abnormal
— Subconjuctival haemorrhages frequently occur following completely normal birth.
— Faintly blue sclera are normal in the newborn so do not assume osteogenesis imperfecta without supporting evidence.
— A newborn term infant should fix, follow and turn to light but may also have a non-paralytic strabismus. This is unusual after 3 months and definitely abnormal after 6 months.
— Congenital ptosis may be unilateral or bilateral and may be associated with inability to look up. Ptosis is not often a sign of myasthaenia in the newborn (unlike the older child).
— The pupils are reactive from 29–32 weeks gestation. Different sized pupils are a normal variant (physiological anisocoria) provided both pupils respond normally to light. A blind eye will show a consensual light reflex but no direct light reflex.
— Each eye may have a different coloured iris (heterochromia-iridia) and this may be a normal variant or a feature of Waardenburg's syndrome.
— If the infant's eyes are open, shine an ophthalmoscope on each eye from about 15 cm away and look for a red reflex. Trying to force his eyes open will make him cry and will not impress the examiners. If the red reflex is absent, or partly obscured, there may be a cataract and formal ophthalmoscopy is indicated at the end of the examination. This involves:
  (i) inspection of the cornea (still from 15 cm away with the ophthalmoscope lens set to 'red 10').
— white cornea and absent red reflex of cataract:
  majority are inherited (usually autosomal dominant)
  intra-uterine rubella

galactosaemia (not present at birth but may appear by second week)

Lowe's syndrome

— hazy broad cornea (>1 cm diameter) of congenital glaucoma. Buphthalmos is tremendous enlargement of the eyeball as an end-stage of the disease:

majority inherited (autosomal recessive)

intra-uterine rubella

— coloboma

CHARGE association:

Coloboma

Heart disease

Atresia choanae

Retarded growth

Genital abnormality or hypogonadism

Ear anomalies and/or deafness

— associated with deformities of the ears and vertebrae (Goldenhar's syndrome).

— conjunctivitis:

viral, bacterial or chlamydial

— dermoid cyst (the eye is a favourite site, usually where the cornea joins the sclera)

(ii) Offer to attempt fundoscopy, although this is unlikely to be taken up unless the infant's pupils have already been dilated with mydriatics. In this case, there is probably one of the following:

— retinopathy of prematurity (retrolental fibroplasia) causing proliferation of new vessels and eventually cicatricial fibrosis and retinal detachment

— chorioretinitis (posterior uveitis) as a result of intrauterine infection

Retinal haemorrhages occur in 20% of all newborns following a normal delivery.

The skull
See Chapter 8. Remember that sutures may be wider or over-riding in the first few days after birth and the anterior fontanelle may be 1–5 cm in diameter. Parietal foramina may occur and are bilateral and familial.

— Fetal scalp electrodes may cause a bruise or small laceration

— caput is pitting oedema and may extend across suture lines

— cephalhaematoma is a tense collection of blood and is bounded by suture lines. Cephalhaematoma should not be confused with cranial meningocoele or encephalomeningocoele. These are usually midline, occipital, soft to palpation, and the bony defect of a cranium bifidum should be apparent

Feel for the reservoir and catheter of a ventriculo-atrial or ventriculo-peritoneal shunt, especially if hydrocephalus is obvious, but leave measurement of the occipito-frontal circumference (OFC) to the end of the examination.

Scaphocephaly is common in 'ex-prems' (up to school age) and plagiocephaly is common and usually benign in term infants.

The mouth   Normal variants:
  (i) Incisor teeth.
  (ii) Epithelial 'pearls' along the midline of the palate.
  (iii) Short lingual frenum (not frenulum which is between upper gum and lip).
    Only very rarely requires surgery for interference with tongue growth or speech.
    Feel along the hard palate with the pulp of your little finger. A cleft palate may be submucous and not visible. Offer to look in the mouth with a bright torch (not an ophthalmoscope which is too dim) and wooden spatula. If the examiners agree to this, there is likely to be one of the following:
  — cleft or soft palate. Look for micrognathia suggesting Pierre Robin sequence. A slanting lower jaw may also reflect intrauterine posture or oligohydramnios (fetal inertia syndrome, in which there may also be talipes equinovarus, camptodactyly and even arthrogryposis).
  — ranula: a cyst in the floor of the mouth arising from the salivary ducts
  — haemangioma of the tongue
  — bifid tongue
  — tongue fasciculation in spinal muscular atrophy (see Ch. 8)
    If there is a white covering of the tongue or buccal mucosa, it may be candida but ask if the infant has just been fed.

The neck   Swellings occurring in the newborn are:
    Midline:
  — goitre
  — thymic cyst
  — thyroglossal duct cyst (moves with tongue movement)
  — epidermoid cyst
    Lateral:
  — sternomastoid 'tumour' (fibrous nodule midway along the muscle which causes torticollis. Usually does not appear until 2 weeks of age and most resolve by 8–10 weeks)
  — cystic hygroma (a benign lymphangioma)
  — branchial cyst (vestigial remnant of branchial arch during ontogeny)
  — ectopic thyroid
    Tumours and abscesses in the neck are extremely rare in the newborn period.

Now undress the baby except for his nappy, always remembering to observe the breathing rate and pattern before disturbing him (see Ch. 5).

The chest	Stridor in the term newborn is most commonly due to laryngomalacia but subglottic stenosis should be considered in an 'ex-prem'. A chronic oxygen requirement is most probably due to bronchopulmonary dysplasia (BPD) and hyperinflation of the chest is a corollary of this. Auscultation gives little information about the respiratory system in the newborn but is usually performed front and back bilaterally while listening to the cardiac sounds.

Feel for both brachial pulses but leave femoral pulses to the end of the examination. Innocent murmurs are much commoner in young babies than older children and the second heart sound is much more difficult to assess.

The hands	Check the palmar creases, count the digits, and look for syndactyly and clinodactyly. Comment on paronychia if present.

The abdomen	This is usually protruberant. Examine the umbilical stump (if present) for:

— infection
— two umbilical arteries
— exomphalos
— granuloma

An umbilical hernia is particularly common in African infants.

Palpate the abdomen in all four quadrants (during which regurgitation frequently occurs and is not abnormal). It is normal to be able to palpate in the newborn:

— tip of the spleen
— 1 cm soft liver edge
— lower poles of both kidneys
— bladder

Leave inspection of the groins, genitalia and hips until the end of the examination.

The nervous system	The commonest pitfall in the neonatal neurological examination is that the responses vary with wakefulness, gestation, and if the head is not in the midline.

1. Cranial nerves: Examination of the face, eyes and tongue has already been described. Most babies will have cried at some point during the above sequence and a feeble cry or persistent irritability and high-pitched cry may be obvious.

— Glabellar tap: a persistent blink response is normal and present from 32–34 weeks gestation.
— Rooting reflex: stroke the cheek and the infant turns his head to that side.
— Sucking reflex: elicited by pressure on the hard palate with a finger while examining for a cleft.

Assessment of hearing and vision are discussed in Chapter 9.

2. Posture: normally flexed 'fetal' or frog-like when supine.

Fully abducted hips in a term infant would suggest hypotonia but the premature infant is normally 'floppy' by comparison. Other features of hypotonia are:

— abnormal head lag
— a tendency to slip through the examiner's grasp in vertical suspension
— a 'rag doll' flexion of the spine in ventral suspension

With arm traction, most term infants have no head lag by 3 months and head lag is definitely abnormal by 5 months. Most term infants maintain a straight back during ventral suspension by 6 weeks. These developmental attainments do not obey postconceptional age, insofar as neurodevelopment is accelerated in the premature infant compared to in utero, but they are still likely to occur at a somewhat later postnatal age than in the term infant.

In the prone position, most term infants cannot maintain 'head up' at 90 until 8–10 weeks. If present at birth, this implies hypertonicity, as does opisthotonus and an extensor posture rather than the flexed 'fetal' posture.

3. Tone and power: These are assessed from resistance to undressing and during assessment of posture.

4. Reflexes: deep tendon reflexes are extremely difficult to elicit in the newborn, except perhaps the knee jerks. Primitive cranial nerve reflexes have been mentioned above. Other primitive reflexes are:

— Grasp reflex: hands and feet in response to pressure. Normally lost by 2 months.
— Stepping reflex: if lowered onto a hard surface. Normally lost by 2 months.
— tonic neck reflex: in response to rotation of the head to one side, the arm on that side extends and the other flexes. Difficult to perform properly as the infant must start in a position with head in midline and limbs held symmetrically. Normally lost by 6 months. An asymmetric tonic neck reflex, say the right arm extends less on rotation of the head to the right than the left arm does on extension of the head to the left, implies an abnormality of the right side in this example.
— Moro reflex: again, must start from a symmetrical position. On dropping the head a few cm, the upper limbs should abduct and extend symmetrically. An asymmetric response again implies a hemiparesis which may be central (e.g. cerebral palsy) or peripheral (e.g. brachial plexus birth injury). Normally lost by 6 months.
— Plantar reflex: bilaterally upgoing until about 12 months.
— Galant reflex: in ventral suspension, stroking one side of the spine causes flexion of the spine on that side. May not disappear until 5 years old.

These reflexes may persist until a slightly later postnatal age in the premature infant but again development is accelerated ahead of the postconceptual age.

Completing the examination

We have suggested that a number of tasks be left until the end of the examination as the child may find them unpleasant. Do not forget to examine, or offer to examine, the following:
1. Femoral pulses.
2. Groins for herniae in either sex.
3. Genitalia:
— increased pigmentation in either sex is abnormal unless Asian or Afro-caribbean baby
— in boys:
    epispadias or hypospadias (glandular, penile or perineal)
    small penis of hypopituitarism
    scrotum for descent of testes and hydrocoeles
— in girls:
    size of clitoris
    labial fusion
    a clear vaginal discharge and blood are both normal in the immediate newborn period
5. Hips (see Ch. 11).
Turn the infant over.
6. Anus, sacrum and spine. Run a finger along the spine, coccyx to occiput. A lumbo-sacral dimple is less likely to be benign if:
— high
— away from midline
— base not visible
— associated hairy naevus or palpable defect in the spine
— weakness of the laegs or patulous anus
7. Occipito-frontal circumference.
8. Fundoscopy.
9. Blood pressure.

Common neonatal long case

The 'ex-prem'

Graduates of the neonatal unit are common and many exhibit persistent stigmata from their admission and some have chronic diseases or handicaps. They therefore make ideal cases for the membership or DCH exams.

History

Great attention must obviously be paid to the history of pregnancy and the perinatal period and most of the pertinent questions have been referred to in earlier chapters (see Ch. 2, 'The long case' and Ch. 8, 'Cerebral palsy'). Detailed questioning is essential about why the infant was born prematurely, if known, and about the exact treatment he received on the

neonatal unit and since. In particular, enquire about the following:
— was immediate resuscitation required in the delivery room?
— did the baby receive oxygen or ventilation and if so, for how long?
— did the baby require a chest drain?
— nasogastric (expressed breast milk or a premature formula) or parenteral nutrition?
— did the baby have one or more lumbar punctures? Why?
— phototherapy or exchange transfusion?

Also try to define the impact of a premature birth on the parents and family. Was the mother transferred in utero or was the baby collected by a 'flying squad'? In either case, the mother may have had to spend long periods away from her kin. Was there a delay before the parents could hold their new baby? Did they 'live in' for a long period and how did they organize transport, work and care of the other children? Did they have fears about death and handicap and do these persist or have they been allayed? What support did they have when the infant was finally allowed home?

Examination   A detailed examination following the guidelines given above must be carried out. Developmental assessment, including vision and hearing, is crucial. The following features are particularly common in infants who have been born prematurely:
— proportionate small stature
— scaphocephaly
— skin stigmata:
    pneumothorax scars
    scars at sites of venous and arterial cannulation
    scars on the heels from repeated 'autolet' stabs
    burns from extravasation of hypertonic fluids (e.g. parenteral nutrition fluids or sodium bicarbonate)
    thoracic or abdominal surgical scars
    bronzing from recent phototherapy
— stridor or tracheostomy following subglottic stenosis
— hyperinflation, recession and tachypnoea of BPD. The infant may still be receiving oxygen by mask or nasal cannulae
— patent ductus arteriosus
— hydrocephalus and/or ventriculo-peritoneal (VP) or ventriculo-atrial (VA) shunt following periventricular haemorrhage. VP shunts block more commonly but VA shunts require more frequent revision as the child grows. Infection rates are about the same.
— retinopathy of prematurity; originally thought to have been explained by excessively high oxygen tension in arterial blood (>15 kPa) but it is now clear that the aetiology is multifactorial.

Discussion You would be expected to be familiar with at least some of the many studies of long term follow-up of low birth weight infants, particularly with reference to:
— neurological development
— physical handicap, including impaired hearing and vision
— chronic lung disease
— sudden infant death

13. Common exam syndromes

The purpose of this chapter is to focus your attention on groups of associated clinical signs which constitute paediatric syndromes. There are many common, and some not so common but characteristic, syndromes which candidates for paediatric postgraduate exams are expected to recognize. There is no substitute for wide clinical experience backed by reference to a comprehensive atlas but an intelligent, logical approach to the dysmorphic child can be practised.

Almost every candidate will encounter a child with a syndrome at some point in their clinical exam. This must be viewed as a chance to score well. If you recognize that a child has William's syndrome and you have been asked to examine the cardiovascular system you should be well on your way to a diagnosis.

In this chapter we have discussed some of the features of some of the more common dysmorphic syndromes which appear in exams with the aim of sharpening your ability to look for associated clinical signs. This is by no means intended to be a comprehensive list, nor have we included all the clinical features of each syndrome.

The dysmorphic neonate The question of whether a neonate is dysmorphic or not is a common clinical problem and one that is sometimes asked in the short cases. When faced with a baby who is 'funny-looking' it is important to have a logical clinical approach. Statements such as 'this baby has low set ears and a degree of hypertelorism' are only acceptable if you can define precisely what you mean, and what measurements you need to make.

In response to the question 'Do you think this is a normal looking baby?', we suggest the following systematic approach.

Cranium:
Is there micro, macro or hydrocephaly present? Offer to measure the maximum head circumference.
Is the shape normal?
Is craniosynostosis present?
Is the occiput flat or prominent?

Eyes:
Is there hypo or hypertelorism? Figure 13.1 illustrates the measurements required to estimate the interpupillary dis-

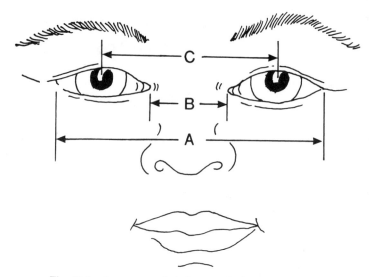

Fig. 13.1 A: outer canthal distance; B: inner canthal distance; C: interpupillary distance — difficult to measure precisely and should therefore be estimated from Figure 13.2 after inner and outer canthal distances have been measured.

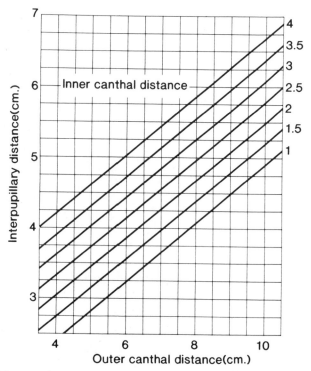

Fig. 13.2 Chart to estimate interpupillary distance from inner and outer canthal distances.

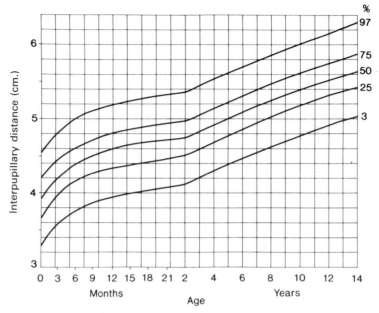

Fig. 13.3 Age-specific norms for interpupillary distance, with key percentiles designated.

tance from Figure 13.2, after which you can refer to Figure 13.3 to determine if there is an abnormality.
Is there microphthalmus?
Are medial epicanthic folds present?
Are the palpebral fissures slanted?
Do the eyebrows extend to the midline?
Are the orbital ridges shallow or prominent?
Is there ptosis of the eyelids?
Are colbomata of the iris present?
Is there corneal clouding or a lens opacity present?
Are the sclerae blue?

Ears:

Are the ears low set? Figure 13.4 describes how to assess if ears are low set. Referral to the appropriate age-related chart, Figure 13.5, once you have determined the percentage of the ear above the eyeline, will determine if a definite abnormality is present.
Are the ears small?
Are the ears malformed?

Face:

Is the face flat, round, broad or triangular? Does the nose look normal?
Is there a low nasal bridge?
Is there malar or maxillary hypoplasia?
ls there micrognathia or prognathia?

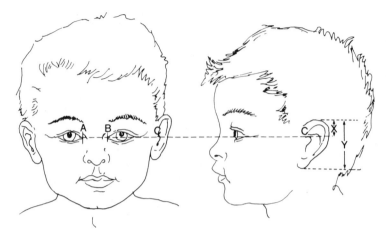

Fig. 13.4 A central horizontal line is drawn through the medial canthi (A and B) an extended laterally to point C where it meets the ear. The percentage of ear above the eyeline is calculated from measurement of X and Y.

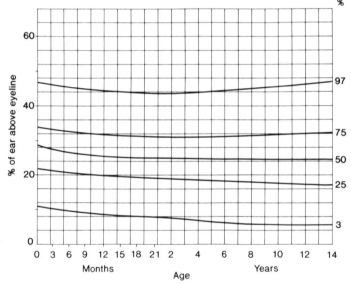

Fig. 13.5 Age-specific norms for percentage of ear above the eyeline.

Is there a cleft of the lip or palate present?
Are the lips prominent or full?
Is macroglossia present?

Hands and limbs:
Is there a single (simian) crease?
Are the hands small with brachydactyly (short fingers)?
Is there clinodactyly (a short in-curved little finger)?

Is there polydactyly (excess digits), arachnodactyly (long fingers) or syndactyly (fusion between digits)?
Are the thumbs and/or toes broad?
Is there aplasia or hypoplasia of the radius?

Skin (see also Ch. 10):
Is there alopecia or hirsutism?
Are there abnormalities of pigmentation?
Is the hair normal?

Genitalia:
Is there hypospadias, micropenis or cryptorchidism?

During your examination it may become immediately apparent that the neonate has a well recognized syndrome, in which case you should search for additional features of the syndrome and demonstrate them to the examiners. If the dysmorphic features do not add up to a syndrome which you recognize, then it becomes important to list the positive and negative findings along the lines described above, so that you would be able to refer at leisure to a suitable reference book.

Neurocutaneous syndromes

These are a group of commonly occurring exam syndromes with classical cutaneous physical signs which should suggest the diagnosis and prompt a clinical search for associated features.

Neurofibromatosis

General

There are two types of neurofibromatosis, type 1 and type 2. Type 1 accounts for over 90% of cases and is inherited as an autosomal dominant with about 50% of cases representing new mutations. Type 2, which is much rarer, is characterized by bilateral acoustic neuromas in over 95% of patients.

Clinical features

Two or more of the following are diagnostic of neurofibromatosis type 1:

1. Six or more café au lait macules >5 mm in greatest diameter in prepubertal individuals and >15 mm in postpubertal individuals.
2. Two or more neurofibromas.
3. Freckling in the axillary or inguinal region.
4. Optic glioma.
5. Two or more Lisch nodules (iris hamartomas).
6. A first degree relative with type 1 by the above criteria.

Associated features and complications:
— Macrocephaly (46% > 97th centile)
— Short stature (34% < 3rd centile)
— Minimal/learning difficulties (30%)
— Scoliosis (11.5%)

— Raised blood pressure (renal artery stenosis [2%] or phaeochromocytomas [3%])
— Malignancy (CNS, optic gliomas; astrocytomas [2%]; other, rhabdomyosarcoma; peripheral nerve malignancy [3%])

Type 2 neurofibromatosis is also associated with café au lait spots but never more than six.

Tuberous sclerosis

General

A syndrome of epilepsy, mental retardation and characteristic hamartomatous lesions which develop in the skin and many other tissues. Inheritance is autosomal dominant with about 86% of cases representing fresh mutations.

Clinical features

Skin. Adenoma sebaceum; fibrous-angiomatous lesions appearing after age 5 years (present in 83%) develop in the naso-labial folds and spread outwards to the cheeks in a butterfly distribution. They vary in colour from flesh to pink to yellow to brown and may coalesce to form firm plaques.

Oval white naevi (depigmented macules) are present from birth in 80% of cases. Periungual and subungual fibromata may appear at puberty. The shagreen patch is usually seen in the presacral region; café au lait patches and pigmented naevi occur less commonly.

CNS. Tuberous hamartomata are present in the cortex and white matter in over 90%, and may calcify. A CT scan of the brain can be diagnostic. Seizures which develop in childhood may be myoclonic or grand mal and are difficult to control. EEG abnormalities are common (87%) and may show a hypsarrhythmic pattern. Mental retardation is common (70%), of whom 100% will develop seizures; of those with average intelligence about 70% will develop epilepsy.

Other tissues.
— Eyes: retinal phakomata (40%); a yellowish, multinodular cystic lesion arising from the disc or retina.
— Heart: rhabdomyomata single or multiple occur.
— Renal: angiomyolipomata (not palpable) in 45–81%, usually multiple, benign and commonly bilateral.
— Lungs: cystic hamartomatous nodules.

Sturge–Weber sequence

Flat facial haemangiomata present from birth, commonly in a trigeminal facial distribution, are associated with haemangiomata of the meninges. The aetiology is unknown, and the condition is associated with grand mal seizures which begin in the first few months and are difficult to control. There may be involvement of the choroid of the eye with glaucoma and bupthalmos. Cerebral calcification may develop and has a classical appearance (double contour).

Short stature   The clinical approach to the child with short stature has been fully discussed in Chapter 7. In this chapter we will discuss some of the more common clinical syndromes which are associated with short stature.

Prader–Willi syndrome   The diagnosis of this syndrome rests on the clinical features, although abnormalities of chromosome 15 have been described in many patients. The common manifestations are short stature, hypotonia in infancy, hypogonadism and mental retardation. After infancy obesity becomes prominent in association with an insatiable appetite, which can cause severe behavioural disturbance in the quest for food.

Clinical features   Facial:
These children have a characteristic facies with a narrow forehead, anti-mongoloid slant to the eyes which are almond shaped, micrognathia and strabismus.

Skeletal:
Small hands and feet, clinodactyly, syndactyly (not polydactyly which is associated with the Laurence–Moon syndrome) and scoliosis are associated.

Neurological:
Mental retardation (IQ 40–70).
Hypotonia in infancy (a history of feeding difficulties is invariable).
Insatiable appetite after infancy.

Endocrine:
Gross obesity.
Hypogonadism: micropenis, hypoplastic scrotum, bilateral cryptorchidism, and in girls delayed menarche. Gonadotropin secretion may be normal or increased.
Diabetes mellitus.

Turner's syndrome   The presence of ovarian dysgenesis, short stature and other dysmorphic features associated with a 45X (or XO) karyotype constitutes the Turner syndrome. It should be excluded by karyotype analysis in all girls who are short and particularly if they exhibit any of the clinical features mentioned below.

Clinical features   Neonatal:
Transient congenital lymphoedema present over the dorsum of the feet.

Facial and skeletal:
A broad thorax with widely spaced nipples, prominent ears, a webbed neck, a high arched palate, a low posterior hairline, a wide carrying angle, a short fourth metacarpal and hyperconvex nails.

Neurological:
Mental retardation is uncommon but a specific defect in space–form perception is often present.

Endocrine:
An increased incidence of auto-immune diseases (particularly hypothyroidism).
Infertility and pubertal failure are the rule due to the presence of streak ovaries.
Short stature is a common problem, the mean adult height being 142.5 cm.

Associated abnormalities:
A high incidence of renal abnormalities, particularly horse-shoe kidneys.
Cardiac defects of which coarctation of the aorta is the commonest.
Excessive pigmented naevi.

Achondroplasia

This is the most common of the skeletal dysplasias of which there are hundreds. If bone disease is suspected as a cause of short stature (usually disproportionate), then a radiological survey of the skull, spine, pelvis and limbs is indicated.

Clinical features:
Megalocephaly
Prominent forehead
Midfacial hypoplasia
Short stature (mean adult height in males is 131 cm and in females is 124 cm)
Short limbs
Thoraco-lumbar kyphosis

Complications:
Hydrocephalus secondary to a narrow foramen magnum
Spinal cord and/or root compression

Russell–Silver syndrome:

This is a syndrome of short stature of prenatal onset with skeletal asymmetry and clinodactyly. Occurrence is usually sporadic and the aetiology is unknown.

Clinical features:
Short stature of prenatal onset
Limb asymmetry
Short incurved fifth finger
Small triangular face
Café au lait spots
Normal intelligence
Bluish sclerae in early infancy

Syndromes associated with cardiovascular lesions (see also Ch. 4)

Down's syndrome	Atrioventricular canal defects
	Patent ductus arteriosus
	Ventricular septal defect

Turner's syndrome	Coarctation of the aorta Aortic valvular stenosis
Noonan's syndrome	Pulmonary valvular stenosis Atrial septal defect
Marfan's syndrome	Prolapsed mitral valve Aortic valve incompetence Dissecting aneurysm of the aorta
William's syndrome	Supravalvular aortic stenosis Peripheral pulmonary artery stenosis Pulmonary valve stenosis
Congenital rubella	Patent ductus arteriosus Ventricular septal defect Peripheral pulmonary artery stenosis
Ellis–Van Creveld syndrome	Atrial septal defect
Holt–Oram syndrome	Atrial septal defect Ventricular septal defect
Maternal collagen disease (e.g. SLE)	Congenital heart block
Pompe's disease Friedreich's ataxia	Hypertrophic obstructive cardiomyopathy
Ehlers–Danlos syndrome	Mitral valve prolapse Tricuspid valve prolapse

This list of associations provides either a clue to cardiac conditions to be excluded if you recognize the syndrome, or alternatively suggests a syndrome diagnosis if, for example, you suspect peripheral pulmonary artery stenosis.

William's syndrome

These children tend to be outgoing and loquacious with a 'cocktail party' personality. The aetiology is unknown but there is an association with hypercalcaemia in infancy.

Clinical features

Facial:
   Prominent lips (and open mouth)
   Medial eyebrow flare
   Short palpebral fissures
   Blue eyes with stellate pattern in the iris

Cardiovascular: (see above)

Neurological:
   Mild microcephaly
   Mild mental retardation (average IQ 56)

Skeletal:
   Mild prenatal growth deficiency
   Hypoplastic nails

Other:
Renal artery stenosis
Bladder diverticula
Partial anodontia

Noonan's syndrome (Bonnevie–Ullrich's syndrome)

Formerly termed the male Turner's syndrome, Noonan's syndrome is associated with a normal karyotype and may occur in both sexes. There is phenotypically some overlap with Turner's syndrome but there are some striking clinical differences.

Clinical features

Facial:
Hypertelorism (75%) (for definition see p. 152)
Anti-mongoloid slant
Epicanthal folds
Ptosis of eyelids
Low posterior hairline
Webbing of neck

Skeletal:
Short stature
Cubitus valgus
Shield chest
Pectus excavatum
Kyphosis/scoliosis

Endocrine:
Males: small penis, cryptorchidism
Females: delayed menarche

Cardiovascular: (see above)

Other:
Renal anomalies are common
IQ is usually below average

The most striking clinical differences between Noonan's syndrome and Turner's syndrome are the presence of mental retardation and right-sided congenital heart disease. The facial features with ocular hypertelorism and down-slanting palpebral fissures are characteristic.

Ellis–Van Creveld syndrome

Clinical features:
Postaxial polydactyly
Micromelic dwarfism (shortening is most marked in the distal half of each limb)
Congenital heart disease (see above)
Ectodermal dysplasia

Inheritance is autosomal recessive.

Holt–Oram syndrome

Clinical features:
Congenital anomalies of the thumb and radius are as-

sociated with atrial or ventricular septal defects. The inheritance is autosomal dominant.

Chromosomal syndromes

Down's syndrome (trisomy 21)

Down's syndrome, which is the commonest autosomal trisomy, is also probably the commonest cause of severe mental retardation. The incidence is approximately 1 in 600 at birth. In our experience a child with Down's syndrome is often present in paediatric examinations. The children are usually very co-operative and enjoy the extra attention lavished upon them. However, as with all things medical, the more common a condition the more you will be expected to know about it. A whole short case may focus, for example, just on the hand in Down's syndrome, so that to score well you need to be well prepared. Many of the clinical features of Down's syndrome are well known and in this chapter we have focused on a few areas which tend to be commonly explored by examiners.

Common features in the newborn

89% of a series of 48 newborns with Down's syndrome had six or more of the following:

Hypotonia	80%
Poor Moro reflex	85%
Hyperflexibility of joints	80%
Excess skin on back of neck	80%
Flat facial profile	90%
Slanted palpebral fissures	80%
Anomalous auricles	60%
Dysplasia of pelvis	70%
Dysplasia of midphalanx of fifth finger	60%
Single palmar crease	45%

The hand in Down's syndrome

Short metacarpals and phalanges (small and broad hands)
Transverse palmar crease (45%)
Fifth finger — Hypoplasia or absence of the middle phalanx (60%)
— Clinodactyly (50%)
— A single crease (40%)
Hyperextensibility
Dermatoglyphics (for an excellent introduction to this important area see Appendix 1 of *Developmental Defects and Syndromes* by M. A. Salmon [HM+M Publishers]).
Palms — distal position of palmar axial triradius
A loop in the hypothenar region (see Fig. 13.6).
A loop in the third interdigital area
Fingers — ulnar loops are common and radial loops may be found on digits IV and V

Common associations

Cataract
Brushfield spots of the iris

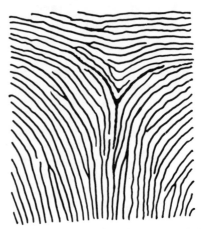

Fig. 13.6 Triradius — the meeting of three dermal ridge patterns. (Reproduced with permission from Forfar J O, Arneil G C (eds) 1984 Textbook of paediatrics, 3rd edn. Churchill Livingstone, Edinburgh.)

Refractive errors
Strabismus

Respiratory disease

Duodenal stenosis or atresia
Pyloric stenosis
Small bowel atresias
Hirschsprung's disease
Anal atresia
Biliary atresia

Hypogonadism and infertility in the male is universal. Delayed menarche, secondary amenorrhoea and premature menopause are common in the female.

Thyroid disorders (more commonly hypothyroidism)
Short stature

Storage disorders

Mucopolysaccharidoses   These are a group of genetically determined disorders of glycosaminoglycan metabolism which are not uncommonly seen in paediatric examinations.

Hurler's syndrome   Poor prognosis with death from cardiorespiratory complications by the end of the first decade. Inheritance is autosomal recessive. Diagnosis is by finding excess secretion of dermatan and heparan sulphates in the urine.
Clinical features:
    Normal appearance at birth

Normal linear growth for the first year followed by the development of short stature
Coarser facies with increasing age
Large tongue and thick lips
Corneal clouding
Retinal pigmentation
Limitation of joint movement with the development of a claw hand deformity
Thoraco-lumbar kyphosis
Hepatosplenomegaly
Hypertrichosis
Intellectual retardation

Hunter's syndrome   Similar features to Hurler's syndrome, but the course is more benign and inheritance is X-linked recessive. There is no corneal clouding. Diagnosis is confirmed by the presence of excess dermatan and heparan sulphates in the urine.

14. The oral examination

In the oral section of the MRCP examination candidates will meet a pair of examiners, each of whom will ask questions for 10 minutes. The examiners are advised to cover at least three and preferably four separate subjects during the 20 minutes. There are a number of areas which examiners are discouraged from exploring, in particular factual recall and data interpretation since these have been tested in the written section of the clinical examination.

Examiners are encouraged to base their assessment of candidates on knowledge of the following:

1. Their understanding of basic principles of physiology, biochemistry, applied anatomy, applied pharmacology and simple statistics.

2. Their ability to manage acute and emergency clinical situations.

3. Their ability to plan investigational and therapeutic regimens for complex clinical problems.

4. Their knowledge of the natural history of diseases.

5. Their ability to recognize, investigate and treat conditions unlikely to be seen in the clinical examination.

6. Their appreciation of social and environmental factors as they affect illness and health.

7. Their appreciation of the importance of communication with patients and their relatives.

It is quite impossible and unrealistic for you to expect to know everything about anything that may be asked in the oral. On the contrary, we would advise you to select topics which you consider a reasonable examiner might *require* you to have a good working knowledge of. For example, we have listed a few subjects which we consider examiners might expect a candidate to have a comprehensive understanding of:

The physiological basis of cyanosis.
The side-effects of long term steroid use.
The causes of hyponatraemia and hyperkalaemia.
The management of an acute asthmatic attack or stridor.
The management of diabetic ketoacidosis.
The investigation of short stature.
The investigation of failure to thrive.
The performance of a sweat test and a jejunal biopsy.

The recommended immunization schedule and established contra-indications. The effect of a chronic illness or bereavement on a family.

These are examples of topics which examiners might reasonably expect a worthy candidate to be able to cope sensibly with. As a rule, most examiners will start the oral with a very general question to which there are no correct answers. One of the authors vividly remembers being asked how to design a neonatal intensive care unit, a question which had never crossed that particular candidate's mind but was clearly lodged in the mind of the examiner who may have been looking for inspiration! If you make a poor start then the examiners are bound to ask you questions that they feel you should be able to answer. Most candidates do not fail on the oral alone; it is the short cases which are at the heart of the exam. However, extra marks can be accumulated in the oral by a well prepared candidate.

Good preparation obviously requires a sound understanding of the kind of topics mentioned above, but also includes a broad knowledge of issues in child health which are currently being debated. The annotations in *Archives of Disease in Childhood* are essential reading. This journal is distributed to all paediatricians who are members of the British Paediatric Association and is thus widely read by examiners. Other useful sources of information include the *Recent Advances in Paediatrics* series and the *British Medical Journal*.

Some useful general advice

Dress smartly; rightly or wrongly examiners expect the candidates to be well turned out.

Treat the examiners with respect and don't look at your feet.

Sit up straight in the chair and do not slouch or fiddle with your hands.

Do not argue with the examiners even if you are certain you are right.

Answer the question asked, and if you don't understand it ask the examiner to repeat it.

Try to think through your answer and frame it in some system of classification before you open your mouth, rather than saying the first thing that comes into your head.

Do not be afraid to say that you don't know. In a sense the examiners want to find out what you do know rather than what you don't. However, if you decline a question which is considered basic, for example the physiological basis of cyanosis, you will not do well!

Don't let yourself become too excited if you are asked something that you are well versed in. The examiners may steer you onto another subject!

Avoid mentioning topics or diseases about which you know

nothing whatsoever; alternatively, you can try to lead the examiners into areas with which you are familiar.

Be prepared for the examiner who asks you what you would like to talk about.

Don't rely on encouraging or discouraging non-verbal clues from the examiners as they are usually not forthcoming.

Do not confabulate!

Appendix: Useful equipment for the clinical examination

Candidates attempting the clinical examination, and especially the short cases, are often unsure of which items of equipment to bring with them. In theory, everything which might conceivably be required should be provided by the examination centre but this equipment will not be as familiar as your own and unnecessary delays may occur while it is located by the exam organisers. There is a need to strike a balance between adequate equipment and pockets which are bulging with everything but the kitchen sink! It is perfectly reasonable to carry a small case or bag with you into the examination containing equipment to aid physical examination and developmental examination.

Essential equipment:

1. Paediatric (not neonatal size) stethoscope with bell and diaphragm.

2. Watch with a second hand.

3. A bright pen torch with fresh batteries which can be used for assessing corneal reflections, papillary reactions and transillumination.

4. Ophthalmoscope with fresh batteries and interchangeable oroscope head. Using an unfamiliar ophthalmoscope or one with weak batteries will not be an asset when you are nervous in the short case situation.

5. Cotton wool.

6. Tape measure.

7. A hat pin with a red head for testing visual fields in an older child.

8. 'Hundreds and thousands' and 'raisins' to test pincer grasp and visual acuity in a young child.

9. A small red cube for testing grasp and visual fixation in a young infant.

10. A small toy which has a rattle (hearing assessment), colour (visual assessment) and which can be grasped by the child.

11. Picture cards (or a book from the 'Ladybird' series) which show:

(a) simple pictures of animals etc. for object recognition or hearing assessment;

(b) situation pictures, e.g. the postman delivering parcels for a child's birthday, to test comprehension and speech.

If the book contains text, make sure you know the appropriate reading age of the material.

This set of aids to the examination should not be assembled the night before the examination. They must be collected and used repeatedly before the examination until you are familiar with the purpose of each item and the age range for which it is appropriate.